JAMES E. LOEHR, Ed.D.

THE NEW
TOUGHNESS
TRAINING
FOR SPORTS

MENTAL, EMOTIONAL, AND PHYSICAL CONDITIONING FROM ONE OF THE WORLD'S PREMIER SPORTS PSYCHOLOGISTS

D0112045

A PLUME BOOK

PLUME
Published by the Penguin Group
Penguin Putnam Inc., 375 Hudson Street, New York, New York 10014, U.S.A.
Penguin Books Ltd, 27 Wrights Lane, London W8 5TZ, England
Penguin Books Australia Ltd, Ringwood, Victoria, Australia
Penguin Books Canada Ltd, 10 Alcorn Avenue, Toronto, Ontario, Canada M4V 3B2
Penguin Books (N.Z.) Ltd, 182–190 Wairau Road, Auckland 10, New Zealand

Penguin Books Ltd, Registered Offices: Harmondsworth, Middlesex, England

Published by Plume, a member of Penguin Putnam Inc.
Previously published in a Dutton edition.

First Plume Printing, November, 1995
20

The Library of Congress has catalogued the Dutton edition as follows:
Loehr, James E.
    The new toughness training for sports : mental, emotional, and physical conditioning
from one of the world's premier sports psychologists / James E. Loehr.
        p.   cm.
    Includes bibliographical references (p. 195).
    ISBN 0-525-93839-7
          0-452-26998-9 (pbk.)
        1. Physical education and training—Psychological aspects.   2. Physical fitness—
Psychological aspects.   3. Stress management.   4. Mental discipline.   I. Title.
GV342.22.L62   1994
796'.01—dc20   94-8921
                                                                                CIP

Printed in the United States of America
Original hardcover design by Steven N. Stathakis

Develop the Flexibility, Responsiveness, Strength, and Resiliency That Is Essential for Success

Toughness has nothing to do with a killer instinct or ruthless play. In *The New Toughness Training for Sports*, sports psychologist and best-selling author Jim Loehr shows how top athletes like Jim Courier, Monica Seles, Ray Mancini, Dan Jansen, and others have benefited from following his emotional, mental, and physical toughness training program. Loehr's groundbreaking techniques are applicable to any sport—individual or team—and provide the essential keys to top performance for both the professional and the amateur.

Praise for James E. Loehr's *Toughness Training for Life*

"Jim Loehr has done it again! His continuing efforts to make us learn more about mental toughness can help people in all walks of life." —Mark H. McCormack, author of *What They Don't Teach You at Harvard Business School*

"Shows us how to get stronger and more productive in life . . . practical tips for people of all ages and interests."
—Stan Smith, U.S. Open and Wimbledon champion, and seven-time Davis Cup winner

"Establishes a 'mind-body connection,' which, when developed, reduces overall stress, increases energy and productivity, improves health, and helps achieve greater happiness from life."
—*Tennis Week*

"Should be required reading for anyone who wants to manage stress effectively." —*Tennis* magazine

JAMES E. LOEHR, ED.D., is president and CEO of LGE Performance Systems, Inc., an Orlando-based research and training facility committed to teaching world-class athletes and high-stress performers how to attain peak performance. Loehr is the bestselling author of eleven books, including *Mental Toughness Training for Sports*, *The Mental Game*, and *Toughness Training for Life* (Plume).

ALSO BY JAMES E. LOEHR

Toughness Training for Life
The Mental Game
Mentally Tough (with Peter J. McLaughlin)
Mental Toughness Training for Sports

To my mother and father, Mary and Con—

For the gift of sport that has added so much richness and dimension to my life.

ACKNOWLEDGMENTS

To Warren and Kitty Jamison for their competence and help in the preparation of this manuscript. To Renate Gaisser for her encouragement and technical skills. To my partners, Jack Groppel and Pat Etcheberry, for their friendship, trust, and support. To Tony Schwartz for his friendship, for his courage to seek personal truth, and for his insights into the Real Self versus the Performer Self. To Tom Dempsey for his vision. To Bob and Vickie Zoellner for believing in the dream. To Gordon Uehling for being the spark.

To the many athletes over the years who have touched my life and made this book possible, who for reasons of confidentiality I do not list here. To mention just a few other special people: Mike, Pat, and Jeff Loehr, Tim and Tom Gullikson, Paul Roetert, Ron Woods, Stan Smith, Irv Dardik, Karen Elsea, Tracey Scolaro, Scott McTeer, Dave Herman, Jan Groppel, Dave Murray, Jackie Point, Dennis Van der Meer, Nick Hall, and Elizabeth Backman.

CONTENTS

FOREWORD BY CHRIS EVERT

Performing well under pressure is what competitive tennis is all about. Many talented players fall short of their dreams because they simply couldn't execute under pressure. As a professional, it became so clear to me that great mechanics, speed, talent, and even fitness were not enough to achieve enduring competitive success.

Although I felt my ground strokes were the best in the game for many years, I didn't possess a killer forehand or knifing volleys. I was certainly blessed with exceptional athletic ability, but I was neither the fastest or the strongest in the game at the time.

So how could I become the number-one player in the world, win 21 Grand Slam titles, and remain ranked in the top of women's tennis for so many years? For me, the answer is what Jim Loehr calls mental and physical toughness.

My weapons were concentration, competitive spirit, confidence, fitness, and poise under pressure. I won because I could compete better. My greatest strength was my toughness.

Even as a young junior I began to realize how competitiveness could be used as a great weapon. From the earliest years, my father ingrained in me the importance of concentration, positive attitude, and emotional strength. He also instilled in me the importance of making competition and all the hard work fun. In Jim Loehr's language, my father was my most important IPS teacher (Ideal Performance State). He laid the foundation of tough thinking and tough acting that eventually became the essential core of my competitive success.

I completely concur with Jim Loehr's belief that competitive toughness is an acquired skill and not an inherited gift. His penetrating insights into how competitive skills are acquired clearly reflect his extensive experience with world-class athletes over many years. Perhaps the most important aspect of Jim's work is its practicality and simplicity. His notions of the real self and performer self, of making waves, of training recovery, of how emotional toughness is both mental and physical, and of the consequences of over- and undertraining are invaluable to athletes at every level of skill.

There are so many books available today on the mental side of sport. Jim's book is in a class by itself. It is a must for any athlete seeking to become a better competitor.

FOREWORD BY DAN JANSEN

I initially began working with Dr. Loehr prior to the 1992 Olympic Games in Albertville. My reason for coming to him was so I could get to the starting line in Albertville with my mind free of the difficult times I had in the 1988 Olympics in Calgary, when my sister, Jane, passed away on the morning of my 500-meter race. As the world witnessed, I fell in both my events, the 500 and 1000 meters.

Although my results in Albertville weren't what I had hoped, we did accomplish what we wanted. I never once thought of Calgary before or during my races.

After 1992, our focus turned to the 1000-meter event. I had been the best in the 500-meter for quite some time, but I had trouble with the 1000-meter mentally.

I didn't enjoy the race and almost came to fear it, and expected to tire in the last 400 meters. With two years of work with Dr. Loehr, I began to win 1000-meter races consistently, and started to "love the 1000-meter" and to look forward to it.

In the 1994 Olympic Games in Lillehammer, Norway, our work together took the ultimate test. A slip in my first race, the 500-meter, cost me a certain gold medal. Four days later would be the last race of my Olympic career, ironically, the 1000-meter.

Our work together paid off. In the 1000-meter event, I won the Olympic gold medal, setting a new world record in the process! I would say we passed that ultimate test!

INTRODUCTION

Tears of joy streamed down my face as I watched Dan Jansen skate a victory lap with his eight-month-old daughter Jane in his arms. The Dan Jansen story was clearly the most compelling and deeply moving of my entire career. Dan began the Toughness Training program outlined in this book on April 23, 1991. From that day forward, until his gold medal performance in the 1000 meters at Lillehammer on February 18, 1994, Dan completed a Toughness Training monitoring log every day of his training life. The goal was simple and straightforward: to leave the past behind and become the best that he could become as a speed skater—at the most important time.

Dan's ten-year quest for the gold is a story of remarkable personal courage and persistence. It is also dramatic evidence of how intimately connected the mind and body are.

The tragic death of his beloved sister on the day of the

xvi   THE NEW TOUGHNESS TRAINING FOR SPORTS

500-meter race at the Calgary Olympics in 1988, his fall in that 500 barely ten seconds into the race, his fall four days later in the 1000, his failure to medal in either the 500 or the 1000 in the Albertville Olympics in 1992, and the loss of the 500 in Lillehammer created what many believed to be insurmountable barriers as he took his final ready position as an Olympian in the 1000. In his last race, with no time remaining on his Olympic clock, in an event he was not supposed to win, Dan Jansen sent a powerful statement to the world:

> It's never over till it's over. Never stop fighting. Never give up. Never surrender. No matter how bad it gets, no matter how deep your pain; persistence, faith in yourself, and an undauntable spirit will eventually break you free.

The story of Dan Jansen is important not as much for his gold medal performance as for what he had to go through to get there. Dan simply showed remarkable toughness through it all. But that toughness was something he trained for everyday. He clearly understood that to summon his full potential at the most important time—with so much adversity surrounding him—required great mental and emotional strength. In the end, it was precisely that inner strength that enabled Dan to triumph.

Building mental and emotional strength is what the New Toughness Training for Sports is all about. My understanding of the process is so much clearer since my first book, *Mental Toughness Training for Sports*, was published in 1986. I am tremendously excited about *The New Toughness Training for Sports* and its companion book, *Toughness Training for Life*, which was published in August of 1993. Both represent quantum leaps in understanding and practical application compared to any of my previous works. The most important breakthroughs are those related to issues of recovery, understanding the language of emotion, markers of overtraining and undertraining, the PERFORMER SELF vs. REAL

SELF, balancing stress and recovery, and the role of awareness in the mental toughening process.

EXACTLY WHAT IS TOUGHNESS TRAINING?

Toughness Training is the art and science of increasing your ability to handle all kinds of stress—physical, mental, and emotional—so that you'll be a more effective competitor. It's a highly sophisticated and thoroughly proven method of perfecting your sport skills while minimizing the risk of physical injuries and emotional setbacks that so often attend overtraining.

A key element in Toughness Training is improving your *recovery-from-stress routines* during practice and between competition. Most sports have recovery periods during play, but many athletes, being unfamiliar with the techniques given here, can't take full advantage of those crucial opportunities for recovery.

Off the field there are equally important recovery demands; for sleep, food, diversion, rest, time off, and so on. Balancing the stress of training and competition with adequate recovery is vital; failing to do so will always undermine an athlete's potential. To achieve that essential balance you have to know how to recognize when you're out of balance. Toughness Training gives you the necessary understandings.

WHAT DOES TOUGHNESS TRAINING TOUGHEN?

Your mind, body, and emotions will become more flexible, responsive, resilient, and stronger—the real meaning of *tough* as used here—through Toughness Training.

How do we do it? Specific exercises for toughening each of the physical, mental, and emotional spheres that make up the whole person appear in several chapters as Toughness Training Assignments. The *New Toughness Training for Sports* gives you an easy understanding of the importance of toughening all three—and shows you how.

You will also learn to recognize overtraining and undertraining, and how to avoid both while keeping your workouts enjoyable and fun. Charts and logs that enable you to track your progress are provided.

The book shows you how to gain access to your Ideal Performance State when you need it most during competition, and shows how to transform your *Performer Self* and your *Real Self* into a powerful, conflict-free partnership that will unlock your competitive potential in a powerful, dynamic way. That's how we do it.

As you will come to discover, Toughness Training is deeply personal and was designed as a very special kind of personal coach. If becoming tougher is your goal, this book will take you as far as you want to go.

THE REAL
MEANING OF
TOUGHNESS

He's very old for an elite athlete: forty-three. Average arms, average legs, no bulging muscles, no definition; in fact, physically he's nothing special. At 155 pounds and 5' 8", he has a walk that is noticeably awkward and flatfooted. Without his glasses he's legally blind. Words like gifted, talented, and genius never come to mind when describing this golfer; terms like average and normal are closer to the mark.

But make no mistake about it, Tom Kite is a one-of-a-kind superstar in professional golf. This very average, nothing-special guy is simply the best of the best in the fiercely competitive world of big-time golf. Tom Kite won the U.S. Open at forty-two and is the all-time leading money-winner in professional golf today. For over twenty years he has mystified his competitors with his precision, consistency, and competitive toughness.

Nothing natural, nothing perfect—just awesome! By his own admission, Tom Kite is an average putter, drives the ball short, possesses marginal mechanics, and is a workaholic. He's even switched back and forth from cross-handed to non–cross-handed putting many times in his career to overcome the yips (hands freezing under intense pressure). And he's not employing some Zen mind-control strategy, not using a secret performance-enhancing drug. So what makes Tom Kite such an awesome competitor? What is his secret weapon? In a word, it's *toughness*!

TALENT, SKILL, OR TOUGHNESS?

To understand the meaning of toughness, you must first grasp the meaning of talent and skill. Everyone has talent—some have it big, some not so big. Talent is genetic potential. It's one of the greatest prizes in Mother Nature's lottery. Athletes can't take credit for it because it's a gift. Theoretically, talent defines the outer limits of your athletic achievement. If you're gifted, a real natural, the idea is that you can be great. However, if Mother Nature's gift was less than generous, the assumption is that nothing special can happen athletically.

Here's where it starts getting confusing. Almost everyone would agree that Tom Kite's talent is nothing special. He's clearly not a natural. But he is the best of the best. Whatever Tom Kite's genetic potential might be (with all the advanced sport science tools available today, reliably measuring talent is still not possible), he has realized it to the fullest. In spite of what appears to be obvious genetic limitation, Kite has become the best professional golfer on the planet. So the idea that talent defines the limits of greatness simply doesn't hold up.

Now let's look at the notion of skill. Whereas talent is a gift, skills are learned. The mechanics of jumping, running, shooting, hitting, and kicking are skills. They are acquired through hard work, repetition, and practice. Theoretically, skills affect achievement in sport in much the same way talent does. Poor physical skills seriously limit potential for success, and great physical skills open it up.

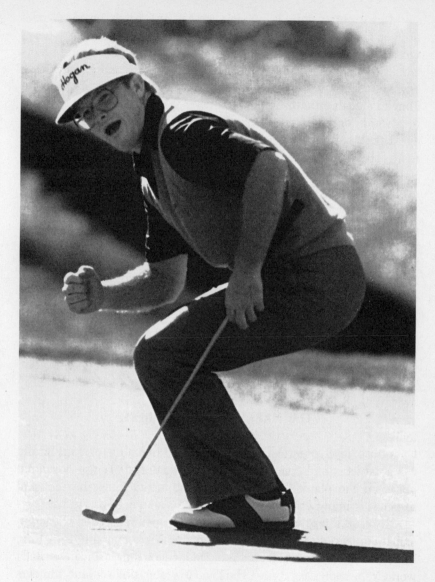

Tom Kite is clearly not the most talented or skilled on the professional tour. He has become the best golfer on the planet because of his competitive skills. Tom Kite gets the most out of what he's got nearly every time he competes. In terms of mental toughness, he has few equals.

But it gets a little confusing again. Tom Kite's physical skills are certainly not the soundest on the professional tour, particularly in the areas of putting and driving. Most of his fellow competitors would rate his mechanical skills between average and good at best. So how does a guy with no special talent and average to good mechanics become the best in the world?

Talent and skill are important contributors to achievement in sport, but they are obviously not the most important factors. So many highly successful athletes exist today who are not gifted or have not achieved mechanical perfection. They're everywhere in every sport—in golf, tennis, baseball, basketball, boxing, skating, hockey, soccer—the list goes on. So what is the critical factor in athletic achievement? The answer is what I call toughness.

I wrote my first book, *Mental Toughness Training for Sports,* nearly twelve years ago. The intervening twelve years of work with athletes at every level of achievement has deepened my understanding of toughness as well as my conviction of its fundamental link to achievement. Now, however, toughness means much more to me than mental. It has become a three-dimensional concept involving physical, mental, and emotional components.

THE MARKERS OF TOUGHNESS

Countless myths persist about the real meaning of toughness. Many athletes and coaches have got it confused. Tough has nothing to do with the killer instinct or being mean. It also has nothing to do with being cold, hard, insensitive, calloused, or ruthless.

Look at the great ones, the lifetime super-achievers: Chris Evert, Jimmy Connors, Michael Jordan, Joe Montana, and Tom Kite, to name only a few. Do words like cold, calloused, insensitive really fit their competitive profile? Hardly. How about words and phrases like flexible, responsive, strong, and resilient under pressure—do these fit better? Without question. What I discovered was that the real markers of toughness are four things:

1. *Emotional Flexibility*—the ability to absorb unexpected emotional turns and remain supple, nondefensive, and balanced, able to summon a wide range of positive emotions (fun, joy, fighting spirit, humor) to the competitive battle. Inflexible athletes are rigid and defensive in emotional crisis and therefore are easily broken. Emotional inflexibility indicates a lack of toughness.

2. *Emotional Responsiveness*—the ability to remain emotionally alive, engaged, and connected under pressure. Responsive competitors are not calloused, withdrawn, or lifeless as the battle rages. Emotional unresponsiveness also reveals a lack of toughness.

3. *Emotional Strength*—the ability to exert and resist great force emotionally under pressure, to sustain a powerful fighting spirit against impossible odds. The inability to fight emotionally is nearly synonymous with a lack of toughness.

4. *Emotional Resiliency*—the ability to take a punch emotionally and bounce back quickly, to recover quickly from disappointments, mistakes, and missed opportunities and jump back into battle fully ready to resume the fight. Slow emotional recovery indicates a lack of toughness.

WHAT TOUGHNESS IS

We now know the markers of toughness, but those still don't tell us what toughness really is. Let's start with a simple definition.

TOUGHNESS IS THE ABILITY TO CONSISTENTLY PERFORM TOWARD THE UPPER RANGE OF YOUR TALENT AND SKILL REGARDLESS OF COMPETITIVE CIRCUMSTANCES.

Although this explanation seems simple enough, a much deeper understanding is necessary before we can move forward. To help you with this, I've expanded the above definition further.

- *TOUGHNESS IS LEARNED.*
  Make no mistake about it: toughness has nothing to do with genetics or inherited instincts. It is acquired in precisely the same way all skills are. If you don't have it, it simply means you haven't learned it. Anyone can learn to get tougher at any stage in his or her life.

- *TOUGHNESS IS THE SKILL THAT ENABLES YOU TO BRING ALL YOUR TALENT AND SKILL TO LIFE ON DEMAND.*
  You may have the talent of a Michael Jordan and the mechanical perfection of a Nick Faldo, but if you don't have toughness, it's as if neither existed. But if you develop great toughness, you can achieve great things regardless of the other two. With toughness you can learn whatever mechanical skills you need, and toughness will push your talent to its absolute limits. Only through toughness can you discover your real limits. Far too many athletes sell themselves short by assuming they are not talented enough. The limiting factor for most athletes is not talent but toughness.

- *TOUGHNESS IS IDEAL PERFORMANCE STATE CONTROL.*
  An Ideal Performance State (IPS) exists for every athlete. It's simply the optimal state of physiological and psychological arousal for performing at your peak. Arousal is reflected in heart rate, muscle tension, brain wave frequency, blood pressure, and a host of other measures. IPS is typically accompanied by a highly distinctive pattern of feelings and emotions—a most fascinating discovery. You are most likely to experience IPS and perform at your peak when you feel:

Confident
Relaxed and calm
Energized with positive emotion
Challenged
Focused and alert
Automatic and instinctive
Ready for fun and enjoyment

- *EMOTIONS RUN THE PERFORMANCE SHOW.*

Make no mistake about it. Emotion runs the show in sport. Some emotions are empowering and free your talent and skill; other emotions are disempowering and effectively lock your potential out. Empowering emotions are those associated with challenge, drive, confidence, determination, positive fight, energy, spirit, persistence, and fun. Disempowering emotions are those associated with feelings of fatigue, helplessness, insecurity, low energy, weakness, fear, and confusion. The reason emotion is so important is its connection to arousal. Emotions are biochemical events in the brain that can lead to a cascade of powerful changes in the body. These changes either move you closer to or further away from your IPS. Fear moves you away, confidence brings you closer; temper and rage move you away, fun and enjoyment bring you back.

- *TOUGHNESS IS THE ABILITY TO CONSISTENTLY ACCESS EMPOWERING EMOTIONS DURING COMPETITION.*

Learning to access empowering emotions during competition, particularly during tough times, is the basis for learning to be a great fighter. That's what toughening is about. *The New Toughness Training for Sports* will teach you how to consistently trigger the right internal emotional climate for maximum competitive success. Emotional control brings bodily control. Roller-coaster emotions produce roller-coaster competitors—lots of ups and downs.

- *TOUGHNESS IS MENTAL, PHYSICAL, AND—ULTIMATELY—EMOTIONAL.*

What you think and visualize, how you act, when and what you eat, the quantity and quality of your sleep and rest, and especially your level of fitness, can all have profound effects on your emotional state at any given time. As you will see, tough thinking, tough acting, fitness, proper rest, and diet are prerequisites for feeling tough. Too many athletes make the mistake of believing that toughness is strictly a mental thing.

■ *IN THE FINAL ANALYSIS, TOUGHNESS IS PHYSICAL.*
This may sound quite shocking coming from a psychologist, but all the evidence is there. The body is physical; talent and skill are physical; emotions are neurochemical events and are therefore physical; and thinking and visualizing are electrochemical events in the brain and are also physical. Athletes make the mistake of believing that what they think, particularly negative thinking, has little effect on their performance. Their notion is that thinking is simply pushing air around inside their head. Since they can't see their thoughts and emotions, they view those thoughts and emotions as not as real or as important as the physical stuff. Well, let's get it straight once and for all: thoughts and feelings are physical stuff too; they are just as real and every bit as fundamental to achievement as talent and skill.

A SOFTWARE-HARDWARE ANALOGY

Analogies can be very helpful in understanding complex concepts. One of my favorite toughness analogies for athletes comes from the world of computers. Just about everyone today knows about computer hardware and software. Software includes all the programs the computer can run, and hardware covers all the mechanical equipment needed to process whatever software programs you use. In the context of sport, talent and skill are the software and the human body is the hardware system required for processing. And just as with computers, you may have the most brilliant software package imaginable, but if the hardware can't process the software, it's as if all that performance potential never existed.

In sport, part of the software theoretically cannot be upgraded or improved because it's genetic (talent). The skill portion of the software, however, can be constantly upgraded and improved. Successful processing of the software requires two things: (1) a well-maintained and healthy hardware system (body) and (2) the proper links between the hardware and software that can carry the current of IPS empowerment.

If the hardware breaks down, or the links between software and hardware break down, the system fails. In the context of sport, this simply means that athletes will be unable to fully access their talent and skill on those competitive days.

And where is toughness in this analogy? Well, it's the most important part. Toughness embodies all the factors that make the links connecting the hardware and software work.

Running an athlete's very sophisticated software requires a very precise kind of current to the software. And the current that empowers the software and brings it to life is *emotional.* As depicted in Figure 1.1, the right current consists of feelings of confidence, challenge, fun, relaxation, positive fight, and determination. Feelings of fear, helplessness, rage, fatigue, depression, discouragement, and low energy either limit access to an athlete's software or shut it down altogether. It's simply the wrong current.

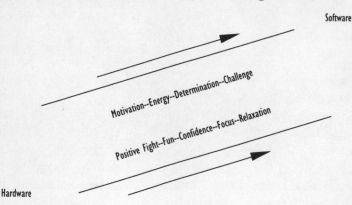

FIGURE 1.1 EMPOWERING CURRENT

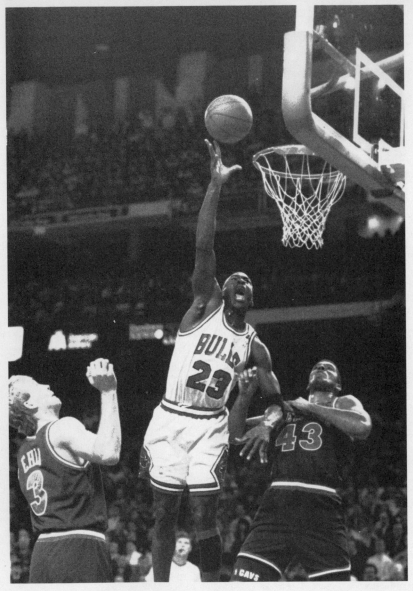

Michael Jordan was cut from his high school basketball team because his coach saw nothing special. He wasn't good enough. How tragic would it have been for him and the world had he responded to the disappointment by quitting. Michael's message is compelling—hang in there. Nobody defines the limits of what you can become but you!

SUMMARY

Never limit yourself by believing you're not talented enough or smart enough, or that you haven't been given the genetic gifts to achieve great heights. Your future is determined far more by what you do than by what you are genetically. The most powerful force in your life as an athlete will clearly be your acquired level of toughness. And the toughness you learn for sport will also prove invaluable to you in the greater arena of life. Everyone needs toughness, and that's what this book is all about.

2

ACCESSING

YOUR

PERFORMER SELF

You learned in Chapter 1 that performing toward the upper range of your talent and skill is directly related to your ability to maintain an Ideal Performance State during competition. Mobilizing your body's performance potential requires a very special kind of psychological and physiological balance. Feelings of relaxation, calmness, high energy, positiveness, alertness, focus, confidence, instinctiveness, determination, and enjoyment form the basis of this delicate state and reflect a very special condition of bodily arousal.

Feelings and emotions simply mirror what's happening deep within your body's physiology. For example, feeling relaxed reflects the amount of electrical energy being transmitted through the muscles of your body. When your muscles feel tight it means a great deal of electrical energy is being delivered, and feeling loose means the opposite.

Feelings of calmness, alertness, and focus reflect a particular pattern of neurological (brain) arousal. Your brain is oscillating at a particular frequency (called EEG) when that special sense of calmness and focus appears. Feeling instinctive and automatic in your play also reflects a special balancing of the right and left hemispheres of your brain.

Feelings of confidence, energy, aggressiveness, and fun reflect a very specific biochemical and neurochemical balance in the body. Feelings of helplessness and fatigue are rooted in opposing biochemical processes. Blood sugar levels, blood sugar stored in the muscle (called glycogen), levels of adrenaline and noradrenaline, and concentrations of special brain hormones (called neurotransmitters and neuropeptides) are just a few of the factors that influence our moment-to-moment feelings and emotions during competition.

When our feelings shift from confident to fearful, powerful changes occur in the brain's chemistry that can profoundly influence coordination and balance, concentration and muscle-response accuracy.

Feelings and emotions, like the instrument gauges of a race car, constantly feed back information about the internal condition of the car's source of power, its engine. These include oil pressure, temperature, RPMs, voltage, and fuel levels. Our feelings and emotions provide similar constant feedback regarding the internal conditions of our bodies and our capacity for continued energy expenditure.

Negative feelings and emotions during competition may point to critical bodily deficiencies that should be immediately tended to, such as the need to consume more cold water to prevent further dehydration or to consume more carbohydrates to raise blood sugar. Negative feelings also confirm that the current flowing between the hardware (body) and software (talent and skill) is contaminated or impeded. The chemistry underlying our negative feelings and emotions can block our efforts to achieve Ideal Performance State *control*. This makes our emotional state during competition crucial to success.

THE PERFORMER SELF VERSUS THE REAL SELF

The way you really feel and the way you need to feel to perform at your best level may be worlds apart. In the context of this Toughness Training System, the way you really feel is called your *Real Self* and the way you need to feel to perform at your peak is called your *Performer Self*. Understanding how the two interact is fundamental to becoming a tough competitor.

Feelings and emotions are flowing all the time, some positive and some negative. Emotions are really body talk carried on by the body's chemical messengers. Positive emotions generally signal balance and health; negative emotions typically signal unmet needs of some kind. *Each and every negative feeling and emotion that we experience serves a purpose.*

Some negative states signal important unmet needs and some signal trivial needs. A child crying because of hunger obviously has an important unmet need; a child crying because his mother won't buy a certain toy sends quite a different message. Similarly, in sport, an athlete feeling low energy and helplessness due to excessive water loss clearly has an important unmet need; throwing a temper tantrum because he failed to score when he had the chance reveals quite another need.

The important thing to understand here is that the body gets its needs met by sending chemical messengers that take the form of feelings and emotions. This brings attention to whatever condition of imbalance exists within the body. Needs can be physical, such as hunger and thirst, or they can be psychological, such as needs for love, recognition, approval, and self-esteem. *Toughness* comes from responding to negative messages in appropriate ways; if you totally block them out, meeting your needs becomes virtually impossible, meaning that your competitive performance will go into a steep decline.

The competitor's dilemma again surfaces here. We know the feelings and emotions we need to feel during competition to perform at our best (IPS) level, but the reality is that what we need to feel may be light-years away from the way we actually feel. Feelings of confidence, high energy, relaxation, enjoyment may never appear at all or suddenly evaporate at the first sign of trouble. Confidence may be replaced with fear, relaxation with tightness, energy with fatigue, enjoyment with frustration or anger—the list goes on and on. Corresponding changes in brain chemistry and physiology accompany these shifts in feelings.

Let's look at some examples of the various ways the Real Self and Performer Self interact.

-------------------- **SITUATION #1** --------------------

Larry is a tennis player. He wins the opening set 6–1 and is ahead 4–3 in the second. He feels and plays great—his IPS is rolling. Although he's winning, the points have been long and grueling and it's very hot. Suddenly Larry starts feeling tired. His concentration falters and he loses the second set 7–5. He loses the first game of the third set and on the changeover becomes acutely aware of his feelings of fatigue, low energy, and reduced confidence. He also acknowledges that the match has consumed nearly two hours already and that it's exceedingly hot.

Larry decides to start taking a liquid carbohydrate sport drink on all the remaining changeovers in the event, believing that his fatigue and tiredness might be due to low blood sugar. He is right. Although he loses the second game of the third set and goes down 2–0, by the third game his energy and confidence start to return. As the third set proceeds, his IPS returns and he wins the third 6–3.

Let's now look at this chain of events in terms of Larry's Real Self and Performer Self. How Larry really felt at any particular point in his match was his Real Self; that is, his psychological and physiological needs were constantly being expressed via his Real Self feelings and emotions. His state of recovery, the condition of his body hardware, his level of fitness, his emotional needs, and his level of self-esteem are all factored in. How Larry needed to feel to perform at his highest level is his Performer Self. This is his IPS and determines whether his hardware (body) and software (talent and skill) will fully connect during match play.

For a set and a half, Larry's Real Self and Performer Self were united. Then declining blood sugar eroded his IPS, eventually preventing him from accessing his Performer Self. Once he became aware of the negative feelings, he responded to the deficiency need by consuming a carbohydrate drink. As his blood sugar rose, his Real Self and Performer Self were reunited and his level of play improved accordingly.

Larry's failure to sustain his IPS during the second set resulted from the following causes:

1. Unmet physical needs associated with his real self
2. Physical demands that exceeded his coping capacity

When the demands of a competitive event approach your physical limits, accessing the Performer Self becomes increasingly more difficult. Unmet physical needs can literally block IPS. As Vince Lombardi observed so often in his lifetime of coaching championship football teams, "Fatigue makes cowards of us all!"

It's important to understand that when the physical demands of a competitive event exceed your capacity for coping, IPS is generally over.

───────────────── SITUATION #2 ─────────────────

Karen enters the race fully prepared physically. She is well rested, has met all her nutritional needs, and has physically trained hard for this all important event. Her parents and friends are present, as well as a few college scouts. Her performance in this race will likely determine whether she gets a college scholarship.

Karen begins the race feeling nervous and tight. She runs considerably below her potential and becomes increasingly negative, frustrated, and angry as the race progresses. When she falls far behind many of her competitors toward the end of the race, her spirit is completely broken and she ceases to try. After the race, she is devastated.

Let's look at what happened. The most important factor is that Karen's Performer Self never became engaged during the race. Feelings of nervousness and frustration dominated the performance. This apparently occurred for psychological reasons. One possible explanation is that Karen's Real Self was simply too needy and unbalanced emotionally to give her access to empowering IPS emotions. The release of stress hormones associated with nervousness and fear could potentially stem from her feelings of insecurity or doubt relative to her running or to more deeply rooted fears associated with generalized low self-esteem.

Another possible explanation for Karen's exaggerated fear response (called choking in sport) is that the emotional demands of the competitive event simply exceeded her coping skills. Pressures from parents, coaches, and college scouts were simply too much.

Karen's failure to achieve her IPS during the race resulted in the following:

1. Unmet emotional needs associated with her real self
2. Emotional demands that exceeded her coping capacity

Just as with unmet physical needs, unmet emotional needs can also block IPS. When the emotional demands of a competitive event exceed one's coping limits, the consequence is loss of IPS control.

SITUATION #3

John plays basketball for his high school team. The winner of this game advances to the finals of the state championships. John is a senior and his dream has always been to play for a state title. He enters the game well prepared physically and emotionally. Most of his physical and psychological needs have been taken care of before the game and he is very fit physically.

Although a little tight and nervous at the start of the game, John eventually settles down and gets his IPS flowing. Midway into the first quarter he is playing well and feels great. Suddenly he is called for traveling on an easy breakaway layup to take the lead. This makes him furious because he feels certain the referee made a mistake. John then commits a foul and a bad defensive error, both of which lead to baskets.

The coach pulls him from the game to settle him down; John interprets this as an unfair slap in the face. When he returns to the game he is noticeably negative and unresponsive, making his disappointment and unhappiness obvious to everyone.

At half time, John's coach publicly chastises John for his lack of toughness. John enters the second half of the game embarrassed and hurt. His negative feelings come through loud and clear in his body language. He is pulled several times in the second half after having played poorly. His team loses the game by eleven points.

Let's take a look at what happened here. Even though John entered the competitive arena well prepared physically and emotionally, and had no serious unmet needs in either realm, he failed to sustain his IPS during almost two-thirds of the game. So what happened? Why did John have such difficulty bringing his Performer Self to life in the most important game of the year?

We must look at John's history to understand the dynamics at work in his case. His past coaches have always viewed him as a *head case*—talented and skilled but a very inconsistent competitor. His coaches usually described him as being wimpy. He constantly whines, complains, and displays negative attitudes. According to his coaches, John wears his emotions on his sleeves, and if he doesn't feel right, he simply can't play. Coaches view John as a good example of a spoiled kid: someone who simply can't tolerate defeats, refusals, disappointments, and all the other inevitable noes of competition and life in the adult world, someone who has a very low tolerance for stress because he's had it too easy. His parents have consistently been accused of overindulging and overprotecting him.

John's failure to sustain his IPS during play resulted essentially from two factors:

1. His poorly developed performer skills
2. His weak and underdeveloped Real Self

In the first case, John's undisciplined ways of thinking and acting under stress make it almost impossible for him to consistently access the emotions that empower him. His failure to learn to think tough and act tough during stressful times makes him vulnerable to every emotional storm that strikes. As you will learn in the next chapter, *tough thinking* and *tough acting* are critical performer skills.

The second cause of John's competitive failures clearly derives from his overprotected and overindulged childhood. Low tolerance for emotional stress, particularly disappointment, hard times, and frustration, frequently results from such an upbringing. Because of his reality-deprived childhood, John simply can't take many emotional hits.

EXPANDING OUR UNDERSTANDING OF TOUGHNESS

This chapter shows that toughness is a multidimensional concept. As we saw with Larry, Karen, and John, the ability to perform consistently under pressure in the upper ranges of their talent and skill required many things.

The first was a physically well-prepared Real Self. When basic needs for food, rest, sleep, water, and so forth are not met, toughness and IPS control quickly become unattainable. The same thing held true emotionally: when their emotional needs were not adequately met before entering the competitive battle, particularly those associated with self-esteem and self-worth, the problems with nerves, self-doubt, frustration, and perceived failure that Karen and John experienced were inevitable.

Another requirement for toughness is a highly developed and skillful Performer Self. The ability to move from the Real Self to the Performer Self on demand calls for precision thinking and acting skills. The exact nature of these performer skills as well as the best way to acquire them will be covered in the next chapter.

The final requirement is the capacity to endure great physical, mental, and emotional stress. *A fundamental component of toughness is physical fitness.* A low tolerance for physical stress typically means the battle will be lost before it begins. Once athletes reach their physical limits, it's like unplugging the computer from its power source. Toughness requires great *physical* flexibility, responsiveness, strength, and resiliency.

The same thing holds true mentally and emotionally. Toughness also requires a great capacity for mental and emotional stress, and great flexibility, responsiveness, strength, and resiliency.

As you will see in later chapters, this capacity is acquired only through exposure to a specific level of stress. Too little stress and overprotection, or too much stress and overstimulation, reduces your capacity for coping effectively with the challenges of competition and life.

The following chapters will provide concrete strategies for achieving all the prerequisites for toughness discussed in this chapter.

3

THE

COMPETITOR

AS ACTOR

It's showtime. The game begins in ten minutes and this one's important. Your coach and team members are counting on you. You'll do anything not to let them down but you're worried, real worried!

You're perfectly clear about how you are supposed to feel to get your IPS rolling, but you're not even close. You've prepared the best you can physically and emotionally, but you just feel lousy. Nothing is right. You didn't sleep well last night and you have a splitting headache. You still feel jet-lagged from the long flight.

Taking off and landing didn't do much to relieve your sinus infection either. Your energy and confidence are just not there. And to add insult to injury, you just called home and got into a fight with your dad over an unexpected low grade in math. Moments before the game, the coach pulls you aside and reiterates how much your team members are counting on you.

"I need the best from you today," he says, and finishes with, "Give me your best." His final words make you cringe.

So what's the answer for you? The whole thing really isn't fair. You're not an excuse-maker but you never chose to feel sick and weak either.

NOBODY CARES

Do you think your coach, the fans, or your teammates care if you have a splitting headache and a sinus infection, or just had a fight with your dad before the game? Not on your life. They couldn't care less about your problems. They care about only one thing: how well you perform.

Let's step back and look at this dilemma from another perspective. Do you think what happened to you in this example ever happens to super-competitors like Michael Jordan, Chris Evert, Wayne Gretzky, and Jimmy Connors? Do you think they always show up for the game feeling motivated, excited, eager, and confident?

If you're not sure of the answer, let me give it to you. The super-competitors are just like you and me—they get tired, burned out, sick, and sore just like everybody else.

So how do they do it? How do they mobilize their Performer Selves and bring to life the emotions that empower them? By what miraculous means do great competitors transform fear into confidence, tiredness into energy, boredom into fun?

Here's how: they learn exceptional performer skills.

THE COMPETITOR AS ACTOR

It hit me like a ton of bricks when I finally made the connection. I was reviewing a research article in a professional journal linking movement of the facial muscles with specific emotional responses such as anger, fear, disgust, and happiness. The study found that professional actors and actresses could stimulate emotion-specific changes in their bodies simply by moving their facial muscles into the direction of the targeted emotion.

The idea that genuine emotional responses could be elicited simply by moving muscles of the face was certainly intriguing. And then I began to think about the whole notion of professional acting.

Why are actors like Jack Nicholson and Julia Roberts so exceptional? After considerable thought I concluded that the great ones are special essentially because they can vividly bring to life emotions called for in a script. Great actors and actresses have somehow learned to move their emotional chemistry in the desired direction *on demand*. The best ones make the emotions real. They really feel grief, sadness, anger, fear, or happiness when the script calls for it, regardless of how they felt before the scene.

Research has confirmed that the physiological changes that occur in the acted-out (faked) emotion are the same as those that occur in spontaneous, genuine emotion. Great actors literally make the faked emotion become real, and that's why they are so believable and powerful.

And how does all this relate to competitive toughness? The answer is simply this: *great competitors are great actors*. They have learned to move their body chemistry in the desired directions just as actors do. But for competitors the script is always the same: IPS. Great competitors have learned to bring to life feelings of confidence, high energy, relaxation, fun, and challenge no matter how they really feel.

BAD ACTORS

Do you think Hollywood directors care if their actors had a tough day before the shoot? What if Julia Roberts has a headache, is tired, had a fight with her husband, feels stressed out, or whatever? Do you think the director really cares?

No way. Just as with coaches, there's only one issue that really counts, and that's performance. Can Julia Roberts bring the script to life? Can she set aside her Real Self and get her Performer Self rolling?

The reason Julia Roberts is such a brilliant actress is that she can consistently move from the way she really feels to the way she is supposed to feel *on demand*. And she is able to convince the audience that the emotions are real.

Bad actors are those who simply can't bring the script to life. They lack the acting skills to be believable. Poor actors are simply those who can't skillfully access the targeted emotions, or who do so in a way that looks phony. There are lots of bad actors in Hollywood.

There are lots of bad actors in sport too. Bad actors in sport are simply athletes who act out whatever emotions they happen to be feeling at the moment, regardless of the script. If they feel tired they show it; if they feel angry, fearful, disappointed, nervous, helpless, whatever—that's what you get.

"I just have to be myself out there. I'm a very spontaneous person, and I just don't like being phony," is how athletes often explain their failure to follow the performance script.

Sure, they all phrase that cop-out a little differently, but the underlying truth is always the same: they lack both the understanding and the skills to make it happen. Their Performer Selves simply aren't skilled enough.

EVERT WAS A SUPREME ACTRESS

Make no mistake about it: Chris Evert was a great actress. She possessed remarkable performer skills. Her ability to act out confidence, determination, fun, and positive fight, *independent of circumstances,* rivaled any of the great actors in Hollywood.

Evert was constantly acting out the script that empowered her. From time to time she may have felt weak, helpless, or nervous, but these or other negative feelings were simply never allowed expression. Since the performance script in sport always remains the same and Evert was very good at following it, she got lots of practice triggering the right emotions. (For Hollywood actors the script is always changing and so is more challenging.)

Unfortunately many poor competitors appear to be following

a novel script with each new competitive battle. Like poor stage or screen actors, they simply can't follow the designated script, so they are forced back on their own version and must suffer the consequences.

The outcome is almost always the same: they fail to fully access their talent and skill. How does this show up on the scoreboard of sport and at the pay window of life? Whenever winning requires their full talent and skill—they lose.

Clearly Evert knew the script and acted it out, over and over again. She had learned this fundamental but very powerful lesson:

EMOTIONS RESPOND MUCH AS MUSCLES DO.
THE ONES YOU STIMULATE THE MOST BECOME
THE STRONGEST AND MOST ACCESSIBLE.

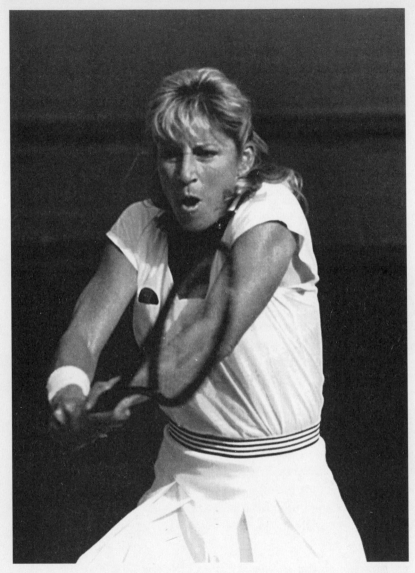

Nobody followed the performance script better than Chris Evert. She was a consummate competitor. Chris's poise, grace under pressure, and fighting spirit brought her genius to life in a dramatic way. In terms of toughness, she was simply the best of the best.

WHAT ARE PERFORMER SKILLS?

How do great actors and actresses trigger specific emotions on demand? Think about that intriguing question. Suppose I offer you $1,000 if you can produce tears of sorrow—onions not allowed. How will you try to do it?

To get the tears flowing and pocket the $1,000 you will likely do two things. First, you will concentrate your thoughts on something very sad in your life: maybe a pet dying, a grandparent passing away, something tragic and gut-wrenching. If you can sustain the concentration long enough, feelings of sorrow and pain will start to break through. However, if you allow your mind to wander, even for a few moments, the sadness will evaporate and so will your chance at the $1,000 prize.

The second thing you can do to help the tears along is to start acting sad with your body. Put on the saddest face possible, even make your chin quiver as it does just before you really cry. Drop your head and shoulders and start breathing in long, broken sobs just the way you do when the tears and the crying take over.

If you're a person who almost never cries, even though you intensively act and think sad thoughts, you probably won't earn the $1,000. The reason is that the crying response is simply too unfamiliar and foreign. However, if you cry easily and if you intensively act and think sad thoughts, you'll probably be depositing the $1,000 in your bank account.

What you have to do to produce genuine tears of sorrow is precisely what actors have to do to bring a script to life emotionally. The skills needed to access targeted emotions are called *performer skills* and generally involve three things:

1. DISCIPLINED THINKING AND IMAGING SKILLS

The thoughts and images you carry in our head have precise emotional consequences. Undisciplined thinking and imaging generally kicks your emotional targets far out of range.

2. DISCIPLINED PHYSICAL ACTING SKILLS

The way you carry your head and shoulders, the look on your face, the way you walk, your body language, also have precise emotional consequences. Acting the way you feel generally intensifies whatever emotion may be present. *Acting the way you want to feel* to achieve your IPS, that is, wearing the mask of confidence, fun, fight, moves you closer to your intended emotional targets.

3. EMOTIONAL RESPONSE PRACTICE

If you're hoping for a new emotional response to the same old problem and you haven't had a chance to practice, the odds are strongly against you. Emotional responses need time and stimulation to grow, just as muscles do. Emotional responses require practice time—the more intense, the better—to entrain the underlying biochemical mechanisms.

PERFORMER SKILLS OF ATHLETES

From an emotional perspective, the actor and the competitive athlete face a similar challenge: to perform to their peak they must fulfill their emotional script on demand. Both must be able to skillfully move from the Real Self to the Performer Self. And the key for both is the development of highly refined performer skills that enable them to genuinely move the chemistry of their bodies in the direction of targeted emotions.

Besides the pressures to win imposed by pride and pocketbook, competitive athletes often face intense pressure from family, friends, and coaches. Heavy as those forces are, they are only the beginning. Add hostile crowds; obnoxious competitors; bad refereeing, perceived or real; cheating; costly mistakes that can be made with mind-wrenching ease; miserable weather; jet lag; stomach upset—an almost endless list of circumstances add immeasurably to the challenge.

To meet that challenge successfully, two acquired skills are essential:

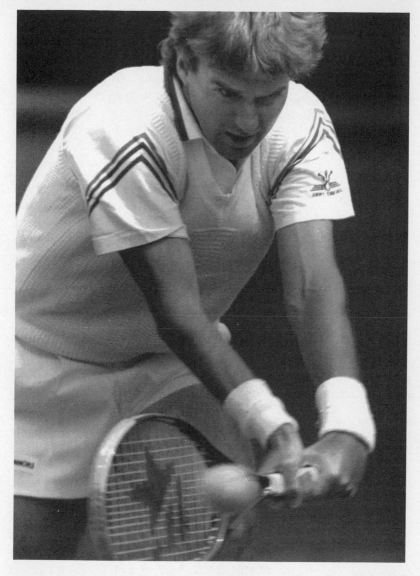

Jimmy Connors is clearly one of the greatest competitors of all time. A supreme actor, Connors was able to powerfully summon feelings of positive fight, challenge, fun and relaxation, regardless of circumstance. His mental-toughness teacher was his mother, Gloria.

I. TOUGH THINKING

This is simply your ability to use words and images to control your Ideal Performance State. This means disciplined thinking and visualization during competition. Tough thinking will keep you from panicking when things get crazy, calm your temper when you make the unthinkable mistake, and prevent you from surrendering when the battle appears lost. Here are some examples of tough thinking.

When the crowd is screaming against you, when you're so tight you can't tie your shoestrings, when all the luck is going the other way—think:

HANG IN THERE, BABY. KEEP FIGHTING.

THINGS WILL TURN MY WAY.

COME ON—I CAN DO THIS!

When old man fear has you by the throat, look him straight in the eye, smile inside, and with all the conviction and passion you can pull from deep within your soul, think—or better yet, say out loud:

I LOVE IT!

When your back is squarely against the wall, think:

THIS IS REALLY TOUGH—BUT I'M

A WHOLE LOT TOUGHER.

When you feel like crawling in a hole and hiding because you're so bad, say to someone in the crowd:

WOULD YOU MIND CALLING 911 FOR ME?

MAYBE THEY CAN BRING ME BACK TO LIFE.

When faced with one problem after another, say to yourself:

> BRING 'EM ON — ALL OF 'EM. IF
> ANYONE NEEDS PRACTICE AT
> SOLVING PROBLEMS, IT'S ME!

When you feel tired, burned out, negative, and weak before the game even starts, think:

> TODAY WILL BE A GREAT CHALLENGE
> FOR ME. I'VE GOT TO BE SUPER-TOUGH
> TODAY TO MAKE IT. IF I CAN DO IT
> HERE AND NOW, I CAN DO IT
> ANYWHERE. I'M GOING TO HANG IN
> THERE NO MATTER WHAT! NO EXCUSES!

When things get painful and you feel like abandoning ship, think:

> I NEVER SURRENDER! NOT ME. NOT EVER.
> I WILL FIGHT UNTIL IT'S OVER,
> AND IT AIN'T OVER TILL IT'S OVER!

When you're playing an opponent you can't stand and your feelings are getting in the way, imagine and believe that you are playing against your best friend, or the person you always seem to play best against.

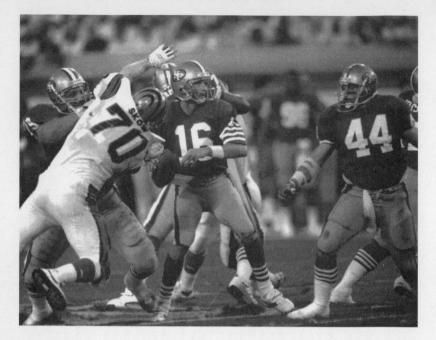

In the eye of the hurricane, Joe Montana remains poised and focused. He will tell you that he literally loves the pressure! Regardless of the odds, Joe believes he can find a way to win. And the tougher it gets, the more he loves it.

2. TOUGH ACTING

This is simply your ability to use your body to control your Ideal Performance State. This means disciplined, precise acting during competition. Like tough thinking, tough acting is a powerful weapon with which to control fear, anger, helplessness, and doubt. Here are some examples:

When you feel your energy and sparkle are gone:

JUMP UP AND DOWN ON YOUR TOES
AND LOOK AS FRESH AS IF YOU'D
JUST ROLLED OUT OF BED ON
THE GREATEST DAY OF YOUR LIFE.

When you make the worst mistake possible:

QUICKLY TURN AWAY FROM THE
MISTAKE AND SHOW NOTHING ON
THE OUTSIDE BUT SUPREME CONFIDENCE.

When the enemy is advancing on all fronts and everyone is panicking:

LOOK AND ACT LIKE A COURAGEOUS
SOLDIER POISED FOR A GREAT BATTLE.
THINK POISE, COURAGE, VICTORY!

When you choked big-time:

BREAK OUT A BIG SMILE AND SEND
THE MESSAGE TO YOUR OPPONENTS
WITH YOUR BODY THAT THIS TIME
THEY WERE LUCKY; NEXT TIME IS YOURS.

When you're down by one with only two seconds remaining on the clock:

MAKE YOUR BODY COME ALIVE WITH THE
MESSAGE THAT YOU LOVE THE CHALLENGE.

When you feel disappointed with yourself or with others:

NEVER SHOW WEAKNESS OR
NEGATIVISM ON THE OUTSIDE.

When the competitive fires burn the hottest:

SIGNAL LOUD AND CLEAR WITH
YOUR BODY THAT YOU LOVE
BEING RIGHT WHERE YOU ARE.
PHYSICALLY RADIATE FUN,
FIGHT, PASSION, AND POISE, NO
MATTER WHAT THE CIRCUMSTANCES.

BELIEVE PASSIONATELY IN THIS SIMPLE
CREED: THE HOTTER THE COMPETITION
AND THE PROBLEMS, THE BETTER!

CAN THE PERFORMER SELF BECOME TOO DOMINANT?

Whenever you're playing a role, the Performer Self is engaged. Most people find it necessary to play a number of roles in their lives. The more roles you must play and the more often you must play them, the fewer chances your Real Self has for expression. It's critical that you distinguish between the acting you and the real you. When acting, you are forcing yourself to conform to a predetermined role so as to achieve a particular goal or objective. When the real you and the performer you happen to end up in the same place by accident, it makes things easy. More often than not, however, you must engage your performer skills to move into the role you need to play. Each time that occurs, some of your Real Self gets pushed aside.

It's a challenging dilemma. If you don't develop and use your performer skills you probably won't accomplish much. Your talent and skill will remain largely untapped. On the other hand, if your

Performer Self dominates your personality, important needs of the Real Self often get suppressed and therefore remain unmet. When the Performer Self dominates someone's personality, a characteristic sense of phoniness and unrealness is often given off. Even among close friends, such individuals project an onstage personality. The real person remains hidden and distant.

The problem with an overly developed Performer Self is that you lose touch with your real feelings and emotions. As you increasingly distance yourself from who you really are and what you really feel and believe, things start getting messier and messier. Important needs go unmet, a sense of alienation sets in, values break down, and things suddenly stop making sense. Your foundation for personal growth, meeting needs, and finding happiness has been eroded. This syndrome certainly infects many in Hollywood. It's seen in sport too, particularly in pro sport.

True toughness in sport requires great balance. A weak Real Self or a weak Performer Self creates imbalance. As you learned in Chapter 2, toughness combines a Real Self that is flexible, responsive, strong, and resilient with a highly skilled Performer Self. The chapters that follow will provide you with new insights and tools to achieve that critical balance.

4

ARE YOU

TOUGH

ENOUGH?

You cannot run away from a weakness;
you must sometimes fight it out or perish;
and if that be so,
why not now, and where you stand.
—Robert Louis Stevenson

Before positive self-change occurs you must recognize the truth and, if what you see is unsatisfactory, accept total responsibility for changing it.

How tough you really are is a big question—the answer that is hammered out on the merciless anvil of competition largely determines how successful you will be in sport. This chapter helps you answer this vital question as accurately and honestly as possible. Wrong answers here bring the entire learning process to a screeching halt.

You bought this book to become a better competitor. Your objective: to get tougher so that you can more consistently perform in competition toward the upper range of your talent and skill.

For that to happen, you've got to come face to face with yourself—no hiding, no protecting, no covering up. In this chapter, you've got to open up the Real Self and take an honest look at what's there. So, for the time being, set aside your Performer Self. Take the mask off—no acting, no pretending. Overcoming this barrier to your competitive success demands a commitment to search out personal truth, to drop the defenses, to take a close, unblinking look at what's really there.

Confronting your weaknesses demands courage; opening up to the truth about yourself can be pretty scary. We spend much energy covering up our weaknesses and very little energy exposing them. Great acting skills are important when we are performing, but they must be set aside to find personal truth.

As you learned earlier, toughness requires both a highly skilled Performer Self and a healthy and balanced Real Self. Chapter 3 explored the performer you, and here we want to explore the real you.

YOUR COMPETITIVE PROFILE

Let's begin the investigative process by completing the Competitive Adjective Profile (CAP)[1] given below. Each item represents a continuum. Try to determine where you think you are on each continuum in terms of your sport; that is, *describe yourself in the context of your sport, not of your life in general.*

Think hard and portray the most accurate picture possible of yourself as you are when you compete in your sport. It's vital to avoid making yourself look a lot better or worse than you really are.

However, being objective about yourself ranges between difficult and impossible. For this reason it's very helpful if three or four

[1] I developed a special version of this Toughness Training Aid for the United States Tennis Association in 1992.

people who know you well competitively also complete the CAP on you. Make sure they understand that you want what they believe is the truth, not what they think you want to hear.

THE COMPETITIVE ADJECTIVE PROFILE (CAP)

10	9	8	7	6	5	4	3	2	1

1. Even-tempered	Moody
2. Resilient (quick emotional recovery)	Nonresilient (slow emotional recovery)
3. Competitive	Noncompetitive
4. Self-reliant	Dependent
5. Committed	Uncommitted
6. Aggressive	Passive
7. Confident	Insecure
8. Patient	Impatient
9. Disciplined	Undisciplined
10. Optimistic	Pessimistic
11. Responsible	Irresponsible
12. Realistic	Unrealistic
13. Challenged	Frightened
14. Coachable	Uncoachable
15. Focused	Unfocused
16. Mature	Immature
17. Motivated	Unmotivated
18. Emotionally flexible	Emotionally rigid
19. Good at problem-solving	Poor at problem-solving
20. Good at team playing	Poor at team playing
21. Willing to take risks	Unwilling to take risks
22. Skilled at acting	Unskilled at acting
23. Strong in body language	Weak in body language
24. Relaxed	Tense
25. Energetic	Nonenergetic
26. Physically fit	Physically unfit

Obviously some of the items relate to Real Self issues and some to Performer Self issues. Any item scored 7 or higher indicates strength. Any item scored 4 or lower indicates weakness.

It's important to understand that the twenty-six performance factors on the CAP are modifiable through training. They do not represent permanent, unchangeable performance factors. Rather, they are acquired patterns of thinking and behaving that affect you emotionally and can have profound consequences on your ability to compete.

WHERE TO START

Under the pressure of competition, we always break at our weakest links. This occurs at every level, mechanically, mentally, physically, and emotionally. If you're a tennis player with a mechanically weak backhand, that's precisely where you will likely break down first as the pressure mounts.

The same thing is true psychologically and physiologically. Faulty patterns of thinking and acting under stress, unhealthy emotional habits, poor physical endurance or strength, and similar weakest links lead to breakdown.

As you learned in Chapter 2, your pattern of weakness eventually disrupts the empowering current flowing between your hardware (body) and your software (talent and skill). Confidence, fun, positive energy, and focus suddenly become fear, doubt, disappointment, and discouragement. And without the current and the chemistry underlying it, you lose the battle fast.

This takes us to one of the fundamental tenets of Toughness Training:

TO GET TOUGHER, ALWAYS FOCUS YOUR
TRAINING ON YOUR WEAKEST LINKS.

It's important, therefore, to know the truth about your weaknesses. That's why feedback from others who know you well can be so valuable. You're simply more likely to get to where you need to start—the *real you*.

No matter who you are, how old or young, how strong or weak, *you can get tougher.* There are only two prerequisites for improving your toughness. First, gain a clear understanding of your weaknesses. Second, develop a strong commitment and strategy for change.

LOW MOTIVATION IS A RED ALERT

Of the twenty-six factors on the CAP, name the most important in terms of competitive success.

The answer is *motivation*. Your level of drive is the number one predictor of how far you will go in your sport. You can improve in all the other factors as long as you're motivated to do so. Take drive out of the formula, however, and the whole competitive learning process collapses.

After completing your profile, first check your motivational score, the only factor where a score below 7 flashes a red alert. Without energy and passion, the current between your hardware and software shuts down; the current that drives all competitive growth and change also shuts down. Beyond its enormous drag effect, what does a low score in motivation mean? Let's assume your motivational score was 4 or 5. This simply reflects the extent to which playing your sport competitively meets important needs for you.

A low score can mean the sport doesn't connect very well with your needs right now. In fact, if you've been performing badly, participation in your sport may actually be keeping important needs from being met. Your needs for recognition, approval, self-esteem, and success can take quite a beating when you're not performing well.

Things can get very lonely, confusing, and painful. And the more you care, the more you hurt when you fail again to make it happen. Athletes figure out very quickly that it hurts less when you don't care as much. As a result, low motivation often becomes a protective strategy for athletes who suffer many perceived failures.

A related cause for low motivation is excessive competitive pressure. The stakes simply become too high. Pressures from overly involved parents, excessively demanding coaches, and other influential people can take all the fun away. Only fear remains—fear of failure, of not measuring up, of looking or feeling stupid.

A temporary drop in motivation can be a response to over-training. As you'll see in later chapters, your motivation provides a very useful barometer of overtraining. Temporary drops in motivation often signal excessive stress and represent the body's attempt to force recovery. If you don't feel like doing much, you probably won't, and that means less stress.

So low motivation can be the result of unmet needs, excessive pressure to perform, too much perceived failure and not enough success, too much overall stress, or not enough recovery. At this point it's important only that you acknowledge your low motivation and commit to trying to understand the reason behind it.

ATTACKING YOUR WEAKNESSES

Let's assume that you've taken the CAP and your four lowest scores are as follows:

Impatient—3
Unskilled at acting—4
Weak in body language—4
Unmotivated—6

We're going to begin the Toughness Training Program by at-tacking your weaknesses. Remember, a score below 7 on motiva-tion is a red alert. Now that you've identified your four weakest areas, let's get started on Toughness Training.

—— **STEP 1: STATE THE WEAKNESSES IN POSITIVE FACTOR FORM** ——

I ' M   V E R Y   P A T I E N T ;   I ' M   A   G R E A T

A C T O R ;   M Y   B O D Y   L A N G U A G E   I S

S T R O N G ;   A N D   I ' M   H I G H L Y   M O T I V A T E D .

——————————— **STEP 2: FOR THE NEXT THIRTY DAYS,** ———————————
——————— **MAKE THOSE FOUR POSITIVE FACTORS THE MOST** ———————
——————— **IMPORTANT THEMES IN YOUR LIFE AS AN ATHLETE** ———————

Put reminders up in your locker, on your bathroom mirror, next to your bed—everywhere you can.

Reorganize your feelings about those four factors with visualization technique. Here's how you do it:

- Write one positive factor on each of four 3 × 5-inch cards.
- Think of some scene where you could enjoy being very patient, being a great actor, and using strong body language, and picture having or enjoying something that motivates you strongly.
- Spend between ten and thirty seconds every morning and every night thinking and feeling each of the four emotional factors you're strengthening. The most effective times are when you first wake up and just before you settle down to sleep.

—— **STEP 3: WRITE A ONE-PAGE SUMMARY OF WHAT YOU WILL DO** ——
— **TO IMPROVE EACH POSITIVE FACTOR OVER THE NEXT THIRTY DAYS** —

That means four one-page personal plans for improvement. Title the four plans as follows:

My Plan for Becoming Patient
My Plan for Becoming a Good Actor
My Plan for Showing Strong Body Language
My Plan for Becoming Highly Motivated

STEP 4: TRACK YOUR PROGRESS DAILY FOR ONE MONTH ──
── ON EACH OF THE FOUR POSITIVE FACTORS ──

Give yourself a "+" for the day if you thought you made improvement, a "0" if nothing happened, and a "–" if you thought you moved backward.

Here is a sample record for the first five days of a month:

day	very patient	skilled at acting	strong in body language	highly motivated
1	+	0	–	0
2	0	–	–	0
3	–	+	0	+
4	+	+	+	+
5	+	0	+	+

── STEP 5: AT THE END OF THIRTY DAYS ──
─ RETAKE THE COMPLETE CAP; AGAIN PROFILE ALL YOUR STRENGTHS ─
── AND WEAKNESSES; THEN SELECT YOUR FOUR WEAKEST AREAS ──
── FOR THE NEXT THIRTY-DAY TOUGHNESS TRAINING CYCLE ──

Hopefully you and your coaches will see positive growth. Depending on how much progress you make in thirty days, you may or may not carry the same themes forward into the next month. If you do have the same theme for more than one month, you must completely rewrite your improvement plan. Also work on intensifying the mental images of your twice-daily two-minute visualization sessions.

HOW TO WRITE YOUR IMPROVEMENT PLAN

Step 3 calls for a one-page summary of the way you are going to improve your weakness. This is precisely the process I follow when I work privately with athletes. I briefly discuss the assignment and ask them to have it ready for the next session. Surprisingly, nearly everyone comes back with a detailed plan of action. With just a little coaching, they are able to describe in considerable detail specific things they can do to improve their weaknesses. I encourage them to be as concrete and practical as possible and let them know that they already possess all the information they need to start the change process. They need only spend quality time to think about the weakness and the answers will come.

I now wish to say the same thing to you. Whether your weaknesses are moodiness, dependency, fear, low energy, tightness, or poor physical fitness, you will have considerable insight into reversing the condition if you will take the time and effort to start piecing together practical answers.

Here are just a few examples of practical suggestions you might come up with in your improvement paragraph.

FOR LOW MOTIVATION

1. Take a temporary break from your sport (if you suspect a contributing cause is too much stress and not enough recovery).
2. Make a deliberate effort to have more fun at practice and at games.
3. If parental pressure causes much of your stress, schedule a discussion with your parents to help them understand how their pressure affects you.
4. Set new and exciting goals for yourself. Set daily goals to keep you focused and long-term goals to keep your spirit engaged.

FOR MOODINESS

1. Reduce negative thinking during practice and competition by refusing to let those thoughts enter your mind; replace negative ideas with positive ideas.
2. Consume carbohydrates more regularly (every one and one half to two hours) if low blood sugar might be a contributing element.

3. Be very tough on yourself when you give in to negative mood swings.
4. Determine that you'll act energetic and positive on the outside even when you start to feel moody. Make a game of fooling everyone around you into believing you're in a great mood.

FOR NONRESILIENCY

1. After a tough mistake or disappointment, repeat to yourself, "I can take a hit; I'm getting more resilient every day."
2. During tough times, think, "No problem—quick recovery!" or "I need adversity to get stronger—I can handle this."
3. After every crisis during competition, look on the outside as if you were never hurt emotionally.
4. When things don't go your way, constantly repeat to yourself, "Keep Fighting."

FOR DEPENDENCY

1. Start taking on more responsibility for all aspects of your sport, such as arranging practice partners, transportation, preparing uniforms and practice gear, and pregame meals.
2. Depend less on your parents to push you to practice and to do your homework; depend more on yourself for the big things as well as the small details of your life.
3. Start thinking more independently. "Come on—here is a terrific opportunity for me to show some leadership."
4. Make a list of all the ways you show dependency regarding your sport. Check the ones you want to change.

BEING NOT TOUGH ENOUGH CAUSES YOU PAIN

As you learned earlier, the ultimate measure of your toughness is the extent to which you can consistently perform toward the upper range of your talent and skill during competition. Another measure, surprisingly, is *pain*.

Let's look at physical toughness first. How do you know when you've exceeded your body's capacity for coping with physical stress? Think about running, weight lifting, or doing push-ups. The closer you get to your absolute limits, the more discomfort you feel. When you clearly exceed your limits, pain hits.

Therefore, if you can sustain a great volume of physical stress without pain, you have acquired a high level of physical toughness. Athletes with poor physical fitness are always hurting or injured. This stems from their being in a constant state of physical overtraining because their bodies have such a low tolerance for physical stress.

What do coaches get from their physically nontough athletes? Constant complaints about how their bodies are always hurting or breaking down. The same holds true both mentally and emotionally: exceeding your capacity for coping mentally or emotionally also results in pain. Psychological pain comes in the form of negative feelings and emotions.

If you're not tough enough mentally and emotionally, it shows as persistent negative thinking and feeling. Just as in the physical realm, athletes suffering from these weaknesses are also in a constant state of mental and emotional overtraining. Because their capacity for coping can't meet the day-to-day psychological demands of their sport, they are always in pain, always complaining, always negative.

Examples of mental and emotional pain include the following:

- Mental and emotional fatigue
- Persistent negative thinking
- Bad moods
- Depression
- Nervousness and anxiety
- Boredom
- Low motivation
- Low enjoyment

- Low self-esteem and confidence
- Burnout
- Feeling defensive and threatened

The more pain you experience mentally, physically, or emotionally, the greater the chance that you simply aren't tough enough. The athlete who enters training camp totally unprepared and unfit offers a good example. All the pain and discomfort felt in the training camp signals overtraining. Constantly exceeding your limits spells big trouble in terms of injuries, broken confidence, and poor performance.

SUMMARY

This chapter discussed several vital issues. The first: how to get a real and honest answer to the question whether you are tough enough. Can you consistently perform toward the upper range of your talent and skill in competition? Are you constantly in pain—physically, mentally, or emotionally?

Another section openly explored your unique pattern of competitive strengths and weaknesses. When you break down, how does it typically happen? Discover your weakest link as a competitor. Do you lack performer skills? Is your Real Self too needy? Are you fit enough physically? Your answers to these questions are fundamental to building new strengths.

Beginning to map out new, practical strategies for overcoming weaknesses provided the final important issue in this chapter. Attacking your weakest links earns the greatest dividends in terms of building toughness.

5

WHY AREN'T
YOU TOUGH
ENOUGH?

Why are some athletes tough and others not? Why do some athletes choke or go crazy with anger in situations where others stay calm and focused?

"Why do I always fold when it's important, at the exact times when many of my opponents always seem to play better?"

To answer these questions, let's explore what might be termed *nontough emotional responses*. You've learned thus far that toughness is the learned capacity to produce a unique emotional response in competition. That emotional response might best be embodied in the word *challenge*. When you're challenged you're positively engaged, mobilized, moving forward. The *challenge feeling* often accompanies feelings of fun, positive fight, confidence, and focus. To consistently *respond with challenge* when things get rough during competition requires great emotional skill.

I like to use the analogy of an archer's target to help athletes understand how the *challenge response* develops in competitors.

Let's look first at the least skillful and most primitive emotional response to the stresses of competition—simply giving up inside, often called tanking in sport. On an archery target, tanking is the ring farthest from the bull's-eye.

Tanking ranges from flat-out quitting to subtle forms of excuse-making. Competitors learn very early that simply not caring as much protects their Real Self from hurt when they lose or don't play well. By withdrawing emotionally from the event, they shield themselves from excessive pain.

Excuse-making is one of the most common forms of tanking. Athletes also use the withdrawal of effort to control their nerves. Competitors soon grasp that reducing emotional involvement and caring reduces their fear and nervousness during play. Here are some examples of tanking:

"If I had really tried I would have won. I just wasn't into it today."
"The coach is such a jerk. I'll never play well with him around."
"I hate this stadium. I never play well here."
"My opponent cheated like crazy. That's why I played so badly."
"It doesn't make any difference if I try—so why should I?"

Tanking is particularly common among athletes who have been labeled gifted or talented. To preserve their image of being talented, athletes create a thousand and one excuses to explain poor performances. The most talented athletes often become the worst head cases precisely for that reason. By not performing well because of head problems, the talented athlete protects his Real Self.

"I performed badly because I didn't try, not because I don't have the talent!"

Although tanking will lessen your pain and reduce your nervousness, it carries a staggering price tag: tankers never fulfill their potential because tanking switches off all current to the software. When you withdraw energy, motivation, or effort, everything starts shutting down, meaning that the battle to bring your talent and skill to life certainly will be lost.

So, for those athletes who tank in any form, the answer to the question of why they are not tough enough is:

THEY FAIL TO GIVE THEIR BEST
EFFORT AND THEN REFUSE TO ACCEPT
FULL RESPONSIBILITY FOR THE OUTCOME.

ANGER

Once you learn to control the tanking response, your next emotional obstacle will be anger and negativism. Although it's one ring closer to the bull's-eye on the archer's target, athletes who fuel their competitive performances with negative emotion never achieve real toughness. Anger, temper, and negativism often serve as misguided attempts to protect the Real Self from pain and, just like tanking, can drive nervousness away. Once that connection is made, the temptation to use negative thinking and emotion to control choking and emotional pain can become powerful.

It's important to note the negativism can flow in two directions, toward self or away from self. Of the two, self-directed anger and negativism disrupt Ideal Performance State control the most, and inflict the greatest damage to the Real Self.

John McEnroe exemplifies an athlete who learned to control his nerves with anger. His rage and negativism, however, were always directed away from himself. Line judges, umpires, camera crews, or spectators always became the object of his fury. Once an athlete turns against himself and turns anger inward, he or she quickly loses the battle.

McEnroe is one of the few world-class athletes in all of sport who achieved great competitive success using the chemistry of anger to control fear. Ninety-nine out of every hundred who follow in his footsteps go up in flames.

McEnroe learned that when he directed his anger away from himself and toward chair umpires, linesmen, opponents, or fans, his nervousness would suddenly subside. And to reduce the potential negative effects of the emotional tirade, McEnroe became very skillful at quieting his anger before starting the next point. To avoid carrying the anger into the next point he would take additional time between points, and perform an elaborate set of rituals that helped him settle down and get his concentration back on track.

Fueling performance with the chemistry of anger is like pouring gasoline on a fire to keep it going. Sometimes you get away with it, but all too often the fire blows up in your face. I strongly believe that John McEnroe never achieved his rightful greatness for precisely this reason.

He was perhaps the greatest talent the game of tennis has ever known, but McEnroe's failure to learn to control his nerves in a more effective way was tragic. His use of anger not only blocked the full realization of his talent, but also steadily eroded his sense of joy and fun in playing. Every match became a war, and war is anything but fun.

Here are some of the ways anger and negativism are used by athletes during competition:

■ *TO PROTECT THE REAL SELF*
When you play badly and are defeated by an inferior competitor it's not because you're less talented but because you *lost it* with temper.

■ *TO REDUCE PRESSURE*
Telling yourself you're stupid, dumb, or brain-dead reduces expectations and helps control nerves.

■ *TO INCREASE AROUSAL*
Athletes learn to use anger and temper to get themselves more activated and stimulated. Anger clearly mobilizes more fighting energy.

■ *TO PREVENT CHOKING*
Anger can definitely overwhelm fear. This gives the athlete a

powerful temptation—made more irresistible by repetition—to blow helplessness and fear away with temper. Nobody likes feeling helpless. Most athletes would gladly trade fear for anger.

- *TO LET EVERYONE WATCHING KNOW YOU'RE REALLY NOT THAT BAD*
  If you don't show disappointment or anger, people will think this is how bad you really are. Again, this is another misguided strategy to protect the Real Self.

From the above examples it's easy to see why so many athletes get off track with negative emotion. Although superior to tanking as a strategy for managing competitive pressure, negative emotions obviously won't take you where you want to go. So, for those athletes who use negativism in any form, the answer to the question why they are not tough enough unmistakably is:

THEY FAIL TO FUEL THEIR COMPETITIVE
FIRES WITH POSITIVE EMOTION.

CHOKING

Once the fear-reducing strategies of tanking and anger are no longer used, athletes come face to face with the choking response. Choking means performing poorly because of fear. Fear unleashes powerful, primitive hormonal responses that can be extremely disruptive to performance. Although fear can completely block talent and skill from expression, it occupies the ring closest to the bull's-eye on the archer's target.

Choking means you're only one ring away—one step away—from where you need to be to perform well. Athletes who choke are clearly tougher and more emotionally skilled than those who either tank or use temper and negativism to cope. Here are some basic truths about choking:

- Everyone chokes sometimes. No matter how tough you get you'll always be vulnerable to choking.
- Choking simply means you care and are engaged emotionally.
- The only sure way to prevent choking is to quit emotionally!
- Toughness means *being able to cope with choking* rather than being able to eliminate it.
- Tough thinking and tough acting will help substantially in controlling the choking response.
- Choking is a biochemical event. The hormones associated with fear are real and so are the effects.
- Choking is not all in your head!

So why do some athletes choke so much more often than others? Why are some athletes so much more vulnerable? Here are some additional insights that are crucial for answering those questions:

1. The more fragile and insecure your Real Self, the more vulnerable you are to choking.
2. Higher confidence lowers the risk of choking.
3. Higher motivation increases the risk of choking.
4. Overly involved parents often enormously increase their children's risk of choking.
5. The more you fear choking, the more you will choke.
6. Learning to control the choking response involves a number of acquired toughness skills.

Choking indicates strength in a very real sense. Choking means you're tough enough to face fear head-on and not back out emotionally with tanking or temper.

It's unfortunate that so many athletes give themselves so much grief for choking and so little grief for tanking or becoming negative. Choking means you're risking and hanging in there. Although you can't always prevent the chemistry of fear from sneaking in, effort and attitude are always within your grasp. The key point is:

ATHLETES WHO CHOKE BUT STILL
CONTINUE TO FIGHT WITH
100 PERCENT EFFORT AND TOTAL
POSITIVISM SHOW GREAT TOUGHNESS.

RISING ABOVE THE PAIN

Choking can be gut-wrenching. During the battle you feel awful; after the battle you feel even worse because you know your talent and skill never became fully engaged. You're often left feeling empty, betrayed, and cheated. Some of the loneliest and most desperate moments for athletes are those that involve choking. That's precisely why you need to fully understand the process.

Mastering the choking response is not unlike learning a complex new physical skill. Before you learn the new desired response, you're going to have to make many wrong responses. Choking is simply the wrong response. But just as when you're learning a new physical skill, if you give up emotionally or become exceedingly negative, you'll never learn the right response.

Learning to control fear takes lots of practice. It is, in fact, the greatest challenge of competitive sport. *Give special attention to this critical understanding: Choking—a completely normal and natural response—in no way reflects personal weakness or frailty. On the contrary, choking means you're closing in on the bull's-eye and often signals that you're developing great emotional bravery.* Confronting fear head-on and refusing to retreat emotionally always demands great courage.

THE CHALLENGE RESPONSE

Getting tough when the heat hits means becoming emotionally challenged. When adversity strikes it means no retreating, no whining, no excusing, no raging. The archer's bull's-eye means hanging in, holding on, mobilizing, firing up, and forging ahead when almost everyone else is heading for the locker room.

Rather than fear and helplessness, what you get is distinct feelings of aggressiveness, spirit, and fight combined with a profound sense of calmness and confidence. Competitive problems become stimulating rather than threatening and—since positive emotion fuels the challenge response—a sense of loving the battle gradually takes form.

To love winning is easy; to love the battle requires toughness, a skill that is honed only through dedicated emotional target practice.

SUMMARY

The answer to the question why you're not tough enough usually comes down to not having learned the thinking and acting skills that make the challenge response a competitive reality for you. To be sure, tanking, anger, and fear are perfectly normal and common responses to the pressures of competition.

Responding to crisis, adversity, and pressure with a sense of challenge and love of the battle is neither common nor normal. Instead it is the mark of the winner, the leader, the champion. Habits of tanking and negativism tragically block the learning process. Only through acquired toughness will this unique and priceless emotional response come within reach.

In the next chapter, we'll explore in further detail why moving beyond tanking and negativism is so difficult for some athletes.

6

WHY CAN'T

YOU TOUGH

IT OUT?

Have you ever broken an arm or leg and had to wear a cast for several weeks? Do you remember what your arm or leg looked like when the cast was removed? You'll probably never forget it. Shriveled up. Scrawny. Weak. Scary. That's a dramatic example of what happens when muscles are overprotected from stress.

The principle is very simple: when muscles are protected from stress they progressively weaken. If the cast stays on for a long time, exposure to even the slightest stress becomes too much for the muscles to handle. Broken bones result from too much stress; deteriorated muscles result from too little stress.

Overstressed bones and understressed muscles react the same way we do when exposed to too much or too little emotional stress. The inability to *tough it out* during competition often springs from a history of either too much or not enough emotional stress. Both emotional overprotection and overexposure can result in competitive problems.

Not surprisingly, parents play a pivotal role in the toughening process in the early years. Chronic problems with tanking, negativism, and choking for young athletes are often linked to parental practices. Parents who push too much, who place too much importance on winning, who live out their dreams through their kids, who withdraw love, affection, and warmth after a failure to perform can create bone-crunching emotional stress.

When traumatized by excessive pressure to perform, the Real Self suffers reduced emotional flexibility, responsiveness, strength, and resiliency. The ability to consistently produce the challenge response during competitive battle requires a healthy, balanced Real Self.

Excessive parental pressure can easily overwhelm the Real Self, causing repeated failures to perform emotionally. Excuse-making, temper tantrums, and choking commonly result. So here's one possible answer to the question *Why aren't you tough enough?*

TOO MUCH STRESS IN THE FORM
OF EXCESSIVE PARENTAL PRESSURE
HAS WEAKENED YOUR REAL SELF.

Although problems with the Real Self are often connected to too much pushing from parents, imbalance can result from any number of other influences as well. As you might expect, however, many of the most powerful Real Self influences are connected to early parental practices.

Parents who consistently fail to meet needs for safety, security, love, and affection also undermine the toughening process. Unfulfilled emotional needs represent powerful sources of stress, particularly for young, developing athletes. The Real Self becomes too needy and fragile to withstand the ego-blows of competition. Losses cut painfully deep: failing to perform devastates self-esteem.

Athletes who carry strong unfulfilled needs for love, affection, and self-esteem into competition consistently find the challenge response out of reach. The psychic stakes are too high for them, the emotional costs of failure too great. Fear of failure becomes the dominating force, and as a result competition becomes too threatening.

So here's a second possible answer to the question *Why aren't you tough enough?*

TOO   MUCH   STRESS   IN   THE   FORM

OF   UNFULFILLED   BASIC   NEEDS   HAS

WEAKENED   YOUR   REAL   SELF.

EMOTIONAL CASTS

Many competitors who lack toughness have clearly been emotionally overprotected. You've seen how too many parental noes in the form of need fulfillment can undermine the toughening process. Too many yeses from parents have precisely the same effect: a weakened, nontough Real Self. Parents who overindulge their children with too many environmental yeses undeniably block the toughening process.

Overprotected, overindulged children are often called spoiled. Spoiled athletes make poor competitors because they truly can't tolerate the stresses of competition. Life has been too easy for them to build emotional strength and resiliency. Just as our muscles require stress to develop and grow, so do our emotions.

Athletes from affluent homes often have trouble in this area. They definitely have had it too easy. Too many environmental yeses create weakness, not toughness. Never hearing *no* outside competition virtually guarantees their inability to withstand competition's relentless barrage of noes. As every real competitor has learned, competition constantly presents noes during play. To respond with challenge when the noes come hard, fast, and heavy requires lots of practice both on and off the athletic field.

Getting tougher for overprotected athletes requires the gradual removal of the emotional cast. This means risking more, putting yourself emotionally on the line more, taking more hits emotionally. It means no more playing it safe. No more running away. No more emotional escapes. It means you've got to stop hiding and face the heat. As soon as you do, the toughening process begins immediately.

So a third possible answer to the question, *Why aren't you tough enough?* goes like this:

TOO LITTLE STRESS IN THE FORM OF
ENVIRONMENTAL NOES HAS RESULTED
IN A WEAKENED REAL SELF.

Obviously it doesn't change a thing merely to learn that you're not sufficiently tough—that your Real Self isn't flexible, responsive, strong, or resilient enough to withstand the pressures of competition. However, understanding *why* moves you a vast distance toward success in the change process. Understanding the influence that parents, coaches, teachers, and others may have on your toughness or lack of it can lead to many important insights and vital breakthroughs.

Although parents play the most decisive role in the toughening process during the early years, you can and must take full responsibility for your physical, mental, and emotional toughness from this day forward. The purpose here most certainly is not to lay blame on parents or anybody else. The objective is to understand the forces that have molded you emotionally, take effective corrective action, and then move on to greater playing success.

Chapter 4's Competitive Adjectives Profile (CAP) presented an effective tool for self-understanding. Most of the factors on the CAP relate to Real Self issues. Facing the truth about yourself is Step 1 and Step 2 in gaining as much understanding as possible of how you got where you are today in terms of emotional toughness. Your first Toughness Training Assignment (in Chapter 4) was to complete the CAP and expose your weaknesses.

Your assignment now is to look at those weaknesses and personally explore the reasons why your Real Self has failed to develop in certain areas.

WEAK PERFORMER SELF

What if your Real Self is relatively healthy and balanced but you continue to have competitive problems? Poor competitive toughness actually stems from two broad-ranging factors. The first is an underdeveloped Real Self, the problem we just explored, and the second is an underdeveloped and underskilled Performer Self. If your Real Self is not the problem and you still can't tough it out, your competitive problems probably stem from inadequate performer skills. Let's take a look.

Poor performer skills fall into three categories:

1. *Poor thinking skills.* This is essentially the inability to trigger targeted emotions through disciplined thinking.
2. *Poor imagery skills.* This is essentially the inability to trigger targeted emotions through imagery.
3. *Poor acting skills.* This is essentially the inability to trigger targeted emotions through disciplined acting with the body.

As you learned in Chapters 2 and 3, consistently gaining access to your Ideal Performance State requires highly refined thinking and acting skills. Athletes who have failed to learn to think tough and act tough won't be able to tough it out when adversity strikes. No matter how balanced and healthy your Real Self may be, if performer skills are weak, the fulfillment of competitive potential will be blocked.

The question to be answered here is why. If your performer skills are underdeveloped, what has stood in the way? Why have you remained so undisciplined in your thinking and acting during competition?

Is it ordinary laziness?

Have you ever really worked on your thinking, visualizing, and acting skills?

What influence have coaches and parents had in this regard? Have they tried to get you to be more disciplined and precise in these areas? Or have you questioned whether these mental and emotional skills are all that important—and therefore not devoted much time and effort to learning them?

I want you to explore these issues as your next Toughness Training Assignment. Your objective: to examine two issues in writing. The first: how well developed are your performer skills? The second: how did you get there? This assignment is particularly important for athletes with weak performer skills.

THE MUST-WIN BATTLE

There is one additional problem I want to discuss in the context of why you can't tough it out, one that relates to both Real Self and Performer Self issues. One of the most common reasons why many athletes fail to tough it out is their tendency to turn against themselves when things go badly. It's almost as if the Real Self and Performer Self split into two nonintegrated parts, one part a punishing, know-it-all criticizer and the other an incompetent, even helpless performer.

The Real Self flagrantly jumps ship and becomes a nightmare critic:

"You're so bad, it's pitiful."
"What's the matter with you?"
"You just can't get it."
"You can't do anything right."
"You're so stupid."

Suddenly there are two battles raging: the one against an external opponent and the internal battle against yourself. Out of nowhere, in the heat of battle, a little voice inside begins a relentless litany of self-criticism.

What was once a unified fighting force against an outside opponent suddenly becomes a divided fight within. A battle that must be waged on two fronts is far more difficult to win.

That's precisely why athletes who constantly bail out on themselves in this way never achieve personal greatness. Launching a vicious attack against yourself is actually a form of mutiny. In a real sense it represents another form of tanking, of avoiding responsibility for what's happening.

Think about it. *You* launch a personal attack against *yourself* because you aren't happy with how *you* are performing. That's a lot of yous! Nobody else is in the mix but you. So who is this guiltless know-it-all judge and jury? It's *you*!

If you have ever played on a team whose members kept turning against one another during tough times, you know the consequences. As soon as team members start attacking each other, the performance potential of the team is locked out. The same thing happens on an individual, personal level.

Take a hard look at the reality: *You* are all you've got. *You* make the mistakes and *you* are responsible for them. *You* are also the only one who can muster courage and strength, who can bring talent and skill to life, who can tough it out.

Toughing it out means hanging in there with yourself; it means staying on the same team, not jumping ship, not bailing out. Treat yourself the way you would your best friend while trying to help him or her perform to the best of his or her ability. Would you ever talk to your best friend the way you talk to yourself? That's probably unthinkable.

If you have this problem, it's time to become your own best friend.

SUMMARY

Several possible answers were explored to the question *Why can't you tough it out?* Performance problems are generally traceable to a weakened Real Self, an underdeveloped Performer Self, or a combination of the two. A weakened Real Self results from exposure to either too much or not enough stress, and, not surprisingly, parents play a central role. An underdeveloped Performer Self results from the failure to learn to be highly disciplined in the way you think and act during play.

Undisciplined, sloppy thinking, visualizing, and behavior completely undermine IPS control. Tough thinking and tough acting are prerequisites for being able to tough it out during competitive battle.

The importance and impact of turning against yourself during competition was also explored. Toughing it out is possible only when the Real Self and Performer Self remain unified and function as a complete team. Winning the battle with yourself is fundamental to competitive success.

TOUGHNESS TRAINING ASSIGNMENT

Write a paper (of at least 750 words) exploring why your Real Self is not tough enough. What have been the forces blocking personal growth for you?

Has there been too much stress or not enough?

What has been the influence of parents, coaches, school, brothers, and sisters on your developing toughness?

Have you had it too easy or too tough?

If excessive pressure (not parent-related) continues to be a problem, where is all that pressure coming from?

If it's entirely self-generated, exactly why is fear of failure potentially so devastating?

What makes your Real Self so fragile, so threatened by failure?

The answers to these questions often come slowly. Significant insights require hard thought and determined effort. You've got to dig, listen, think, feel, talk, go away, and then come back and dig again. Facing personal truth and then understanding it is a lifetime journey of fundamental importance to personal growth.

Your goal in reading this book is to accelerate growth in competitive toughness, so the understanding you seek obviously is sport-related. But it's exciting to know that as you grow in emotional flexibility, responsiveness, strength, and resiliency for sport, you grow in your capacity to manage stress in every arena. In a real sense, personal battles won on the athletic field pave the way for even greater victories within the context of life itself. When sport can be used to increase your toughness for life, the payoff is enormous!

TOUGHNESS TRAINING ASSIGNMENT

Prepare a 250- to 300-word summary addressing why you aren't more disciplined in your thinking, imaging, and acting skills during competition. Although your answers will not come easily, the potential insights can powerfully influence your growth as a competitor.

7

UNDERSTANDING
STRESS AND
RECOVERY

In Chapter 6 you learned that either too much or too little stress will undermine the toughening process. Here you'll learn that getting tougher is fundamentally linked to two specific abilities. If you don't already possess these abilities, you can develop them. They are:

1. *Your ability to balance stress and recovery in your training as well as in the broader arena of your life.*
   As you will see, entering battle fully recovered is essential for being a great fighter.
2. *Your ability to generate as many waves of stress and recovery as possible in the area you wish to toughen.*

As you will also see, physical, mental, or emotional toughening occurs as a direct consequence of *making waves,* a concept originally formulated by Dr. Irv Dardik in his hypothetical model of wave energy theory. His application of wave theory to disease reversal provided many insights into the stress/recovery relationship.

To fully understand how stress and recovery relate to the toughening process, we need some working definitions. In the Toughness Training context, stress is anything that causes energy to be expended; recovery is anything that causes energy to be recaptured.

Physical stress occurs when you expend energy in moving muscles; mental stress happens when you expend energy in thinking and concentrating; emotional stress comes when you expend energy in feeling fear, anger, and other emotions.

Physical stress is running a race; mental stress is thinking about race tactics; emotional stress is worrying about how you're going to do in the race.

Recovery occurs at three levels as well—physical, mental, and emotional. Recovery often simply means rest. When you rest, you temporarily break episodes of stress and allow energy to be restored.

Reducing muscle stimulation represents *physical recovery;* breaking concentration and reducing mental stimulation represents *mental recovery;* replacing negative feelings of anger and fear with positive feelings of calmness and confidence represents *emotional recovery.*

Stress and recovery are also closely connected to need fulfillment. Unfulfilled needs represent cycles of stress; fulfillment of those needs is recovery. Likewise, feelings of hunger, tiredness, fear, and depression represent stress; relief from those feelings is recovery.

BALANCING YOUR ENERGY CHECKBOOK

A great analogy for understanding the relationship between stress and recovery is the necessity of keeping your bank account in balance. Stress is spending money; recovery is making deposits.

Most people love to spend money by writing checks, but find that making deposits in their bank account is somewhat more difficult. Nevertheless, it has to be done—if you write checks for more money than you have deposited, you're headed for serious trouble.

In sport, expending more energy than you recover also has serious consequences. In the physical world of sport, chronic failure to balance your energy checkbook leads to muscle failure, exhaustion, and injury. In the mental world of sport, the consequences of expend/recover imbalance are failures to focus, concentrate, or solve problems. In the emotional world of sport, the consequences of expend/recover imbalance are negativism and burnout. In all three areas, imbalance leads directly to victories by opponents who otherwise would have been defeated.

Another useful analogy for understanding stress and recovery is the operation of an electric car. Recharging the batteries allows the electric car to be driven at top speed. However, as the car barrels down the highway, the energy stored in the batteries is consumed. As the batteries approach exhaustion, the electric car slows and all its systems start to fail. Regardless of how brilliant the car's operating potential was with full batteries, once the stored energy is used up the car grinds to a halt; its potential is frozen until energy is recaptured.

Here are some important stress/recovery insights related to toughening:

- Stress is anything that causes energy to be expended; it occurs physically, mentally, and emotionally.
- Recovery is anything that causes energy to be recaptured; it occurs physically, mentally, and emotionally.
- Unfulfilled needs represent forms of stress.
- Fulfillment of needs is recovery.
- In order to fight great battles in competition, your energy deposits should be roughly equal to your energy withdrawals. Your goal should be to enter battle fully recovered whenever possible.
- Balancing stress and recovery is fundamental to becoming a tough competitor.

STRESS AND RECOVERY EXAMPLES

In order to balance your energy checkbook, it's important that you clearly understand when you are expending energy and when you are recovering it. The chart below lists common examples of various kinds of stress; the chart on the bottom of the page lists common examples of recovery.

PHYSICAL STRESS	MENTAL STRESS	EMOTIONAL STRESS
Running	Thinking	Feeling angry
Hitting	Concentrating	Feeling fearful
Jumping	Focusing	Feeling sad
Weight lifting	Visualizing	Feeling depressed
Walking	Imaging	Feeling negative
Moving	Analyzing	Feeling frustrated
Exercising	Problem-solving	Feeling hurt

As mentioned earlier, unfulfilled physical, mental, and emotional needs of the Real Self—needs for food, water, sleep, rest, safety, belonging, self-esteem, self-worth, and recognition—are important sources of stress. The more intense or urgent the need, the greater the stress. Negative feelings and emotions are often linked to unfulfilled needs of some kind.

PHYSICAL RECOVERY	MENTAL RECOVERY	EMOTIONAL RECOVERY
Feelings of bodily relief (reduced hunger, thirst, sleepiness, etc.)	Feelings of mental relief	Feelings of emotional relief
Eating	Increasing calmness	Increasing positive feelings
Drinking	Increasing sense of slowing down mentally	Decreasing fear and anger
Sleeping	Increasing fantasy	Increasing fun and enjoyment
Napping	Decreasing focus	Increasing feelings of safety and security
Heart rate slowing down	Increasing creativity	Increasing feelings of self-esteem

| Breath rate slowing down | Increasing spontaneous imagery | Increasing feelings of personal fulfillment |
| Muscle tension decreasing (feeling more physically relaxed) | Brain activity slowing down | |

Learn to recognize when you are experiencing stress as opposed to recovery. We tend to think of physical stress as being unmistakable, as in swimming a hard training session's last lap. Mental and emotional stress can be somewhat more subtle, as when you can't doze off while trying to take a needed nap because you're worried about not knowing a certain play well enough for tomorrow's game. Being able to distinguish between stress and recovery is extremely important.

Athletes have little chance of finding and maintaining stress/recovery balance without such understanding.

HOW MAKING WAVES PROMOTES TOUGHENING

Let's briefly go back to the example of the broken arm or leg set in a cast. The cast ensures a prolonged cycle of recovery for the broken bone by protecting it from physical stress. Because of the severe damage to the bone, a lengthy cycle of recovery is necessary for the bone to repair itself. For healing to occur, a massive dose of stress (which caused the bone to break) must be followed by a massive dose of recovery.

Completely protecting the arm or leg from stress clearly leads to strengthening of the broken bone. But what about the muscles surrounding the bone that were not injured? As was discussed earlier, the protected muscles start to weaken almost immediately. The lack of exposure to stress caused the healthy muscles to steadily weaken. Eventually, the once healthy muscles will completely lose their capacity for energy expenditure (stress).

What happens to a muscle when it is confined in a cast is not unlike what happens to us when we are overprotected from stress

mentally or emotionally. Being cut off from stress mentally or emotionally is like taking a prolonged vacation.

When the vacation is too long, when we remove ourselves too
long from competitive stress, school stress, training stress, we
gradually lose our capacity for coping with stress in that area. As
we learned in the case of serious injury or trauma (broken bone),
a lengthy vacation from physical stress may be necessary for healing to occur.

This applies to all three areas—physical, mental, and emotional. A serious break mentally or emotionally may actually require
a prolonged recovery period (relief from stress). In the absence of
acute, traumatic injury, however, growth and toughening occur in
response to intermittent waves of stress and recovery. In other
words—wave-making.

The first thing a physician will do after removing a cast from
an arm is to place the arm in a sling. The sling continues to provide
protection for the weakened muscles and bone but allows considerably more stimulation (stress) than the cast. The physician will in-
struct the patient to remove his or her arm from the sling for short
periods (stress) and then return the weakened arm to the sling (recovery).

Rehabilitation of the muscles requires progressively increasing
the exposure to stress and progressively decreasing the exposure
to recovery. Here is a brief summary of how wave-making relates
to toughening:

- Great weakness resulting from serious injury physically, mentally, or emotionally typically requires a prolonged recovery
  time for healing immediately after the injury and then gradual
  exposure to progressively increasing episodes of stress for
  toughening to occur.
- Great weakness resulting from prolonged recovery (too much
  protection) physically, mentally, or emotionally requires gradual
  exposure to progressively increasing episodes of stress for
  toughening to occur.
- Converting physical, mental, or emotional weaknesses into

strengths always means exposure to increasing stress followed by strong waves of recovery. This is precisely what is meant by making waves.

EXAMPLES OF WAVE-MAKING

It's always easiest to understand how things work in the physical world, so we'll begin there.

PHYSICAL WAVE-MAKING

WEIGHT LIFTING TO INCREASE MUSCLE STRENGTH

Doing leg curls, arm curls, bench presses, sit-ups, and so on represents stress; the time between sets of exercises represents recovery. Increasing stress and decreasing recovery times, if done properly, will lead to toughening.

Most weight lifters alternate workout days with rest days to provide a twenty-four-hour recovery period between doses of stress. Lifting weights stimulates growth in the muscles, but your muscles actually grow during recovery.

RUNNING A MARATHON

Running continuously for twenty-six miles represents a powerful dose of physical stress that must be followed by an equally powerful dose of physical recovery, often lasting several days or even weeks.

For the body to withstand the volume of stress generated in a marathon and not break down with injury or exhaustion, the body must be exposed to progressively increasing doses of running stress spread over several weeks. Toughening is evidenced in both faster running times (the ability to tolerate higher volume of stress) and faster recovery times (the ability to recapture lost energy at a faster rate).

MEETING YOUR PHYSICAL NEEDS

Hunger reflects a bodily need and represents a cycle of stress. Fulfillment of the need by eating is recovery. The more the meal meets the body's nutritional needs, the more powerful the cycle of recovery. The same is true for sleep. The need for sleep is stress, and fulfillment of the need by sleeping is recovery. The greater the need for sleep, the greater the stress; the longer and deeper the sleep, the more profound the recovery.

MENTAL WAVE-MAKING

CONCENTRATING DURING PRACTICE

Focusing your attention on a target is stress; allowing your mind to wander is recovery. Many sports require intense concentration over long periods. This capacity for mental work must be built with the same basic system that you use to strengthen muscles—by progressively exposing yourself to increasing stress.

Begin by focusing attention intensely for short periods, followed by recovery. Gradually extend the length of concentration (the volume of stress) and decrease the nonconcentrating time (the time allowed for recovery). This is precisely why concentration during practice is so important to success during competition.

FORMULATING NEW MENTAL HABITS (TOUGH THINKING)

Mental practice, such as visualizing, rehearsing tactics and strategies, and training yourself to think more positively, all represent cycles of stress. Not thinking about such things, not practicing mentally, is recovery.

Most athletes fail to create enough mental training stress. They simply do not practice enough mentally (expose themselves to mental practice stress). As a consequence, they can't sustain the mental work necessary to perform at their peak during competition. Their thinking is undisciplined, unfocused, and nonproductive during play because they consistently failed to generate sufficient mental stress during practice. Like the physical game, the mental game is largely won or lost in the practice weeks that precede play.

MENTAL WAVES DURING BATTLE

A lapse in concentration during competition represents a wave of recovery that can have many negative consequences for performance. Fumbles, double-faults, mistakes of all kinds occur when we lose focus.

These lapses are unplanned recovery waves that often occur during prolonged cycles of high stress. When athletes train to better use mental recovery opportunities that naturally occur during play, unplanned lapses tend to decrease.

An example is the between-point time in tennis. Playing the point demands precise concentration (mental stress); the twenty-five-second period between points represents a great opportunity for a brief recovery wave.

Taking full advantage of recovery opportunities that naturally exist within a specific sport can make all the difference in terms of managing mental stress. Constantly thinking or talking about your sport prolongs the cycle of mental stress and increases the risk of mental lapses at the wrong times.

Mental recovery for a golfer might be playing tennis; for a tennis player it might be playing golf. Changing sports completely breaks normal habits of thinking and thereby creates a valuable recovery wave.

EMOTIONAL WAVE-MAKING

DURING TOUGH EMOTIONAL TIMES, PUT FUN INTO YOUR SCHEDULE

Bad losses, slumps, and missed opportunities all represent potentially powerful sources of stress. Going to movies, hanging out with friends who make you laugh, sightseeing, shopping, anything you can do to have fun creates waves of emotional recovery. Making emotional waves is critical for coping with a high volume of emotional stress.

TO GET EMOTIONALLY TOUGHER, YOU MUST STEP INTO THE FIRE AND THEN JUMP OUT BEFORE YOU
GET BURNED

The fire is the pressure, the fear of losing, the doubt and un-
certainty of competition. If you never take the emotional risk of
stepping into the fire, emotional strength will never come. Stepping
into the fire (emotional stress) and jumping out of the fire (emotional recovery) is the only toughening formula that works.

Recovery is a powerful message sent to yourself: you're still
okay; the loss didn't destroy you; you can take the heat and not get
burned. But to get those messages sent, you must find effective
ways to stimulate emotional recovery.

TALKING STIMULATES EMOTIONAL RECOVERY

Most athletes find that talking about their emotional pain and
inner turmoil with people who care (coaches, family, friends) brings
powerful relief. Locking emotions up inside has precisely the opposite effect. Making waves emotionally generally means moving
from negative to positive feelings and emotions. Activities that can
bring emotional relief and recovery include writing, painting, listening to or playing music, exercise, and meditation.

HOW DO YOU KNOW YOU'RE IN BALANCE?

Depending on what phase of toughening you happen to be in, you
may be expending more energy than you've taken in or you may be
recovering more energy than you are expending. At any given moment in your training, you are likely to be in a temporary state of
stress/recovery imbalance. That's all part of the toughening sequence.

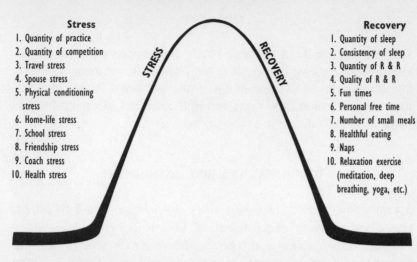

Stress
1. Quantity of practice
2. Quantity of competition
3. Travel stress
4. Spouse stress
5. Physical conditioning
   stress
6. Home-life stress
7. School stress
8. Friendship stress
9. Coach stress
10. Health stress

Recovery
1. Quantity of sleep
2. Consistency of sleep
3. Quantity of R & R
4. Quality of R & R
5. Fun times
6. Personal free time
7. Number of small meals
8. Healthful eating
9. Naps
10. Relaxation exercise
    (meditation, deep
    breathing, yoga, etc.)

FIGURE 7.1 BIG-PICTURE BALANCE

The critical factor is the big picture—how closely your recovery balances your stress over time. It's like your checkbook: you can temporarily write more checks than you have money in the bank as long as you make a deposit before the checks bounce. In terms of the big picture, stress and recovery must be in balance. In other words, total energy out (stress) must be at least equal to total energy in (recovery) or the body will be forced to start shutting down many of its performance systems. Figure 7.1 shows big-picture balance.

The best barometer for determining your stress/recovery big-picture balance is your level of energy. If you feel lots of energy, motivation, drive, and passion, you're probably in great balance. Fun is another great indicator of balance. If playing your sport continues to be great fun, your stress/recovery checkbook should be in good shape.

In the next chapter we'll take a much closer look at the markers of imbalance.

SUMMARY

This chapter explored the way stress and recovery pertain to the toughening process. Getting tougher physically, mentally, and emotionally was linked to the concept of making waves. Markers of balance were discussed and reviewed in the context of having fun and staying motivated.

TOUGHNESS TRAINING ASSIGNMENT

It's now time to do a stress/recovery check. Completing the stress check and recovery check questionnaires will deepen your understanding of how stress and recovery interact daily and weekly. See the Appendix for the forms you are to complete. Fill out the information daily for seven consecutive days and then add up your scores for the week. Instructions for completing and interpreting the results are also provided in the Appendix.

OVERTRAINING

AND

UNDERTRAINING

It's early morning and every muscle in your body is sore and stiff. You hurt all over. Your body's on fire. You're tired, you're cranky, and you hate the world. You've had enough of your coach and his fall training camp. Rolling out of bed and going back into practice sounds like the very last thing you'd want to do.

The coach is determined to get your team in shape—and it's only the fifth day of training camp. You're not the only one who's hurting. Yesterday morning your best friend at camp woke up in a foul mood and flatly refused to get up. The shouting match with the coach that followed ended with your friend exiting the team.

You know it'll be tougher now with your friend gone and nobody left to share your gripes with. Your physical tiredness and soreness carries over into the mental—instead of feeling bright and alert, you feel down and dull. Emotionally you're a wreck because now you have to go through the rest of camp alone.

You know that coaches always put their athletes through hell during preseason training, but somehow you thought the fires of hell didn't burn quite so viciously hot. Ahead of you stretches an endless course of 50-yard dashes, 100-yard dashes, distance runs, wind sprints, sit-ups, push-ups, weight training—you really wonder if you can make it through another day.

This is an example of overtraining. The volume of stress simply exceeds your body's capacity for recovery. And the reason for the overtraining is that your training stress before training camp was not high enough to handle the volume of stress during camp.

All the pain signals one of two things—either you weren't tough enough going into camp or the camp is simply unreasonable. Almost a third of the athletes are taking the regimen in stride, so the problem seems to rest squarely on your shoulders.

You're paying the price for coming into camp seriously undertrained. In the spring, when you signed up for fall camp, you were in good shape, but you took the summer off and did nothing to stay that way; all through summer you dreaded the idea of get-

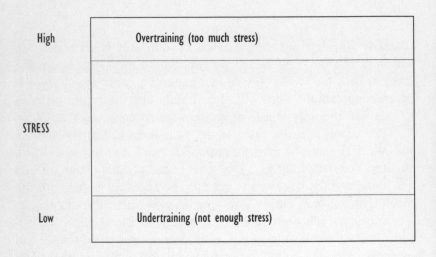

Figure 8.1 The Continuum of Stress

ting ready for fall training instead of doing it. As a result you've entered a very serious period of physical overtraining.

When that happens the body lets you know through soreness—through pain. The markers of overtraining physically are generally unmistakable. This is also a very high-risk period for injuries—shin splints, muscle pulls, groin pulls, calf pulls, cramping.

In the previous example, you entered training camp *under*trained and, as a result, you were seriously *over*trained during camp. Overtraining occurs when the volume of stress—physical, mental, or emotional—exceeds the limit of what you can handle. That limit is called your *adaptation threshold.*

Undertraining occurs when the volume of stress is insufficient for the desired adaptation to take place. And, as you have undoubtedly discovered, the consequence of exceeding your adaptation limit is pain.

Overtraining and undertraining actually represent opposite ends of the same stress continuum. As seen in Figure 8.1, overtraining is too much stress on one extreme and undertraining is too little stress on the other. Both are conditions of imbalance and have distinct performance consequences.

Another way of conceptualizing overtraining and undertraining is in terms of recovery. Undertraining is too much recovery and overtraining is not enough recovery (see Figure 8.2).

In Chapter 7 you learned about making waves, which simply meant alternating cycles of stress and recovery. The opposite of making waves is *linearity.* To be linear simply means to function in a straight line.

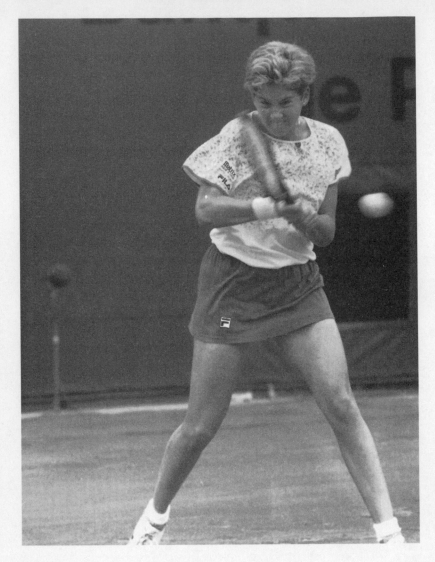

Monica Seles showed exceptional toughness as early as 11 years old. In all my work spanning nearly 20 years, I never witnessed anyone with her capacity for hard work, concentration, and drive at such a young age. Monica's greatness was clearly evident by age 12.

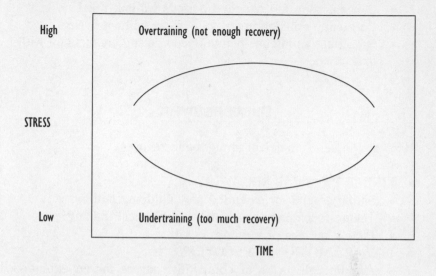

Figure 8.2 Overtraining and Undertraining

LINEAR STRESS

Here are some examples of straight-line stress:

- LINEAR PHYSICAL STRESS
  - Running a marathon
  - Practicing your sport for long periods without breaks
  - Doing any type of steady-state aerobic exercise for extended periods
- LINEAR EMOTIONAL STRESS
  - Worrying about a game or tournament for several hours or days without relief
  - Feeling constant parental pressure to succeed without relief
  - Feeling negative and frustrated for extended periods without relief

- LINEAR MENTAL STRESS
  - Concentrating for extended periods without relief
  - Constantly thinking about your sport without breaks
  - Sustaining an intense mental focus during competition without breaks

LINEAR RECOVERY

Here are some examples of straight-line recovery:

- LINEAR PHYSICAL RECOVERY
  - Sitting around for extended periods doing nothing
  - Taking a complete break from all physical training
  - Putting an arm or leg into a cast
- LINEAR EMOTIONAL RECOVERY
  - Avoiding all forms of competitive stress for an extended period
  - Quitting the team because your coach puts too much pressure on you
  - Never taking risks emotionally
- LINEAR MENTAL RECOVERY
  - Not thinking or focusing about your sport for extended periods
  - Allowing your mind to wander away from competition for extended periods
  - Watching TV for extended periods

THE CONSEQUENCES OF IMBALANCE

Too much stress leads to overtraining and too much recovery leads to undertraining. Surprisingly, both are signaled by pain. The reason for the same pain is that if you're seriously undertrained, you're constantly in the state of overtraining. The pain is actually stemming from overtraining in both cases.

It's critical that you recognize and understand the body's messages of over- and undertraining. The body is always talking through feelings and emotions. Athletes who wish to move to the next level of toughness—physically, mentally, or emotionally—must expose themselves to additional stress. Understanding the body's language of stress and recovery is fundamental to positive growth. Here are some common signals of over- and undertraining.

PHYSICAL	EMOTIONAL	MENTAL
Chronic fatigue	Boredom	Confused thinking
Muscle soreness	Depression	Poor concentration
Injuries	Sadness	Persistent mental mistakes
Constant illness	Low motivation	
Aches and pains	Anger	Chronic mental fatigue
Eating problems	Moodiness	Irrational thinking
Sleeping problems	Anxiety	Poor problem-solving
Weight problems	Lack of enjoyment	Negative thinking

Perhaps the two most important consequences of overtraining and undertraining are that (1) you typically perform well below your potential and (2) rather than getting tougher, you get progressively weaker. Both undertraining and overtraining result in decreasing toughness.

You should also understand:

- Excessive physical stress will lead to mental and emotional problems.
- Excessive emotional stress will lead to mental and physical problems.
- Low motivation, low energy, and fatigue often reflect the body's way of protecting itself against further overtraining.
- Depression, moodiness, and negative emotion serve the same purpose as physical pain.
- Persistent problems with concentration, negative thinking, and nervousness often reflect stress/recovery problems.

- Sleeping and eating problems are common consequences of overtraining.

STRESS THAT TOUGHENS

You now understand that too much stress or too much recovery will lead to progressive weakening. You also know that physical, mental, or emotional pain is the language of over- and undertraining. The question now is, how can you distinguish between stress that toughens and stress that weakens? To answer this you need to look at the issue of stress a little more closely.

As seen in Figure 8.3, the volume of stress can be divided into four categories relative to toughening:

1. Undertraining—too little stress
2. Overtraining—too much stress
3. Maintenance training—too little stress (at this level of stress you will simply maintain your current level of toughness)
4. Toughness training—the volume of stress that leads to toughening (this is called *adaptive stress*)

It's important to understand that only one relatively narrow band of training stress among the four categories leads to toughening. One of the four merely allows you to hold on to your present level of toughness; the other two result in weakening. So the critical question now is how can you tell if the training stress you're experiencing—physically, mentally, or emotionally—is adaptive and therefore toughening, or not?

Figure 8.3 provides the answer. The key is in the distinction between pain and discomfort. To toughen you have to go beyond your normal limits, beyond your realm of comfort. When you simply do what is comfortable in your training you're either getting weaker or maintaining your current toughness level. You clearly have to challenge yourself beyond your normal limits to grow. While you have to cross new frontiers, you must not venture out

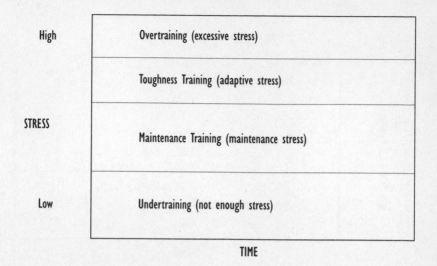

Figure 8.3 Distinguishing Stress that Toughens from All Other Kinds

too far or overtraining will result. There's always discomfort because it's further than you've gone before. The point is simply this:

NO DISCOMFORT—NO TOUGHENING

NO PUSHING—NO TOUGHENING

NO PERSONAL CONFRONTATION—NO TOUGHENING

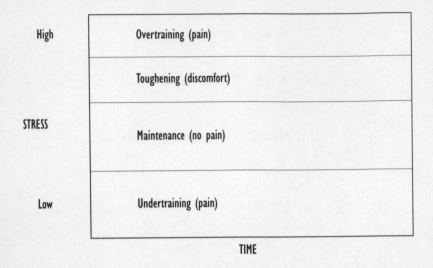

Figure 8.4 The Language of Stress

The objective is to deliberately seek out new challenges in your areas of greatest weakness. Deliberately seeking out stress and pushing yourself to new limits and new frontiers is *active toughening*. Using the uninvited, random challenging stresses of everyday life to toughen yourself is *passive toughening*. In either case, discomfort indicates adaptive stress.

As stated earlier, stress creates the conditions for growth. Recovery is when you grow. Entering the narrow band of toughening stress also creates some stress/recovery imbalance. A short-term imbalance is necessary for toughening to occur. Persistent, chronic imbalance always results in overtraining and progressive weakening.

THE NO-PAIN, NO-GAIN NONSENSE

The "no pain, no gain" ethic is tragically misguided. Pain should be immediately recognized and understood by athletes, be it physical, mental, or emotional.

PAIN IS A SIGNAL TO STOP.
DISCOMFORT IS A SIGNAL TO PAY ATTENTION.

Understanding the way pain is communicated and the way it differs from the discomfort of toughening stress is vital. That's precisely why athletes must be so tuned in to their bodies, their mental states, and their feelings and emotions. And the better-trained and more finely tuned the athlete, the more important it is to accurately decipher the body's stress/recovery messages. Know your markers of overtraining. Know what is too much and learn to say no when you've reached it. Also learn to recognize and tolerate the discomfort associated with—and essential to—toughening stress.

Two basic principles are vital in your training:

1. Never follow the no-pain, no-gain nonsense.
2. When the fun stops, pain is probably not far behind—pay attention!

It's important also to recognize that cycles of stress not accompanied by feelings of either discomfort or pain represent maintenance stress. When you merely do what is comfortable you either get weaker or, at best, maintain whatever level of toughness you already have. The point is you've got to become a good listener, you've got to be able to accurately interpret what you hear, and you've got to learn to respond appropriately.

Highly experienced exercisers learn to tolerate a high degree of discomfort and generally understand when real pain starts and the normal grind of toughening stress ends. What is pain to one person may be discomfort to another. The critical factor is that you know your body and fully understand and remain sensitive to the stress/recovery messages it is sending.

WHERE IS THE IPS?

The question where your Ideal Performance State is on the continuum of stress is an important one. Let's go back to the way you feel when you're performing at your absolute peak. Do you feel pain? Absolutely not. Do you feel discomfort? Not really. When they are "zoning," athletes usually report feelings of effortlessness, challenge, and fun. They do not feel pushed beyond their normal limits even though they may be performing well beyond normal levels. Based on peak performance reports, IPS occurs toward the upper range of maintenance stress. Figure 8.5 shows this.

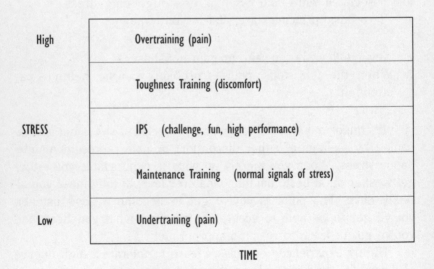

High	Overtraining (pain)
STRESS	Toughness Training (discomfort)
	IPS (challenge, fun, high performance)
	Maintenance Training (normal signals of stress)
Low	Undertraining (pain)

TIME

Figure 8.5 IPS on the Continuum of Stress

HOW MUCH STRESS IS ENOUGH?

Let's assume you can comfortably handle 100 units of physical, mental, and emotional stress. Let's also assume that to stay at your current level of performance, you never need to exceed 90 units of stress. Given these circumstances, you're theoretically tough enough. You simply have to continue to expose yourself to a minimum of 100 units of stress to achieve your objectives.

But what if you want to move to a higher level of performance—say a 3:59 mile as opposed to a 4:10 mile, or a 2:20 marathon time as opposed to 2:45? When you try to achieve these new higher levels of performance with your current level of toughness, you simply get too much pain. The pain has a purpose: it lets you know that you're not tough enough, that you need more training stress.

To achieve your new goals in the mile or marathon, you will have to gradually increase your training stress to 110 or 120 units.

What are the consequences of cutting back your training stress to only 50 units per day after you have maintained 100 units for several weeks?

Before long, your capacity to sustain stress will decline to 50.

If your sport typically requires 90 units and you have been training with no more than 50, the consequences are all too familiar: you never reach your IPS, you deliver no peak performances, you set no new records, personal or otherwise. What you are likely to get is breakdown, discomfort, pain, and perhaps injury.

It's also very important to understand that if you're very tough, you must maintain a very high volume of stress or you'll lose your exceptional capacity to be tough during competition. Once you've reached a high level of physical, mental, and emotional toughness you've got to constantly work to maintain it or you'll simply lose it. Never forget:

TOUGHNESS IS NOT A DESTINATION;
IT'S A JOURNEY WITHOUT END.

SUMMARY

Without stress you simply cannot achieve your goals as an athlete. Finding the balance between too much and not enough stress is a constant, must-win battle if you are to reach your full potential. Learning to distinguish stress that toughens, referred to as adaptive stress, from stress that weakens is a critical athletic skill. The meaning of pain, the role of discomfort, and the importance of fun represent serious training considerations. The no-pain, no-gain rule of thumb has no place in the context of responsible training. To toughen you must break new barriers, but pain simply signals you've gone too far. Avoiding the consequences of overtraining and undertraining not only is a journey without end, it's one of the greatest challenges of sport.

9

TRAINING

RECOVERY

We all understand what training stress means. To coaches and athletes, that's precisely what athletic training is all about. Skillfully administering controlled doses of stress leads to improvement and growth—to becoming faster, stronger, more efficient. However, the concept of training recovery is very new for most athletes.

After intensive study of tennis players who have achieved great success, it became clear to me that recovery skill is one of the most important factors separating frequent winners from consistent losers.

Studying *during*-point time gave very few clues to the essential difference between great tennis competitors—those who were mentally tough—and those who were not. The real insight came when I began to study *between*-point time.

However, I had to study between-point time intensely before the significant differences surfaced and gradually became clear. Slowly I came to understand that this nonplaying time represents a very special recovery opportunity for top competitors. By contrast, poor competitors often throw away the same opportunity.

Highly successful competitors in tennis, I found, go through four distinct phases between points as a trained recovery sequence.

FIRST STAGE: THE POSITIVE PHYSICAL RESPONSE

As soon as a point ends, top competitors show a very strong physical presence. After a mistake, they project the message "no problem" with their body. For many, the look is that of a soldier in battle—fearless, in control, unaffected by adversity.

This positive acting period, we came to understand, was a learned pattern of behavior that served to prevent negative emotions from intruding and contaminating the twenty-five-second recovery opportunity. The positive physical response stage—as it was eventually called—is the launching pad for the Performer Self.

Rather than acting as they really feel at the end of each point— tired, upset, angry, or disappointed—top competitors immediately begin acting in ways that enhance the flow of positive emotion during the recovery period. By comparison, poor competitors typically are much less skillful in following their IPS script during the first phase.

Many were simply bad actors, with the result that the cycle of stress would continue unabated through the entire twenty-five-second interval. The longer the episodes of bad acting, the more linear the match would be in terms of stress.

I was fascinated to discover that top tennis competitors are very skillful at making waves under pressure. Heart rates climb during point and then decline as much as twenty beats between points. This nonlinear, wavelike interaction between stress and recovery clearly is connected to performing well. The more I studied and analyzed the data, the more obvious it became that skillful Stage 1 actors and actresses made the best competitors because they were in fact the best wave-makers.

Although this vital positive physical response stage lasts only three to five seconds, it provides sufficient time to send powerful messages back to the Real Self that everything is under control. No reason to panic, no reason to go crazy with anger.

A distinct pattern emerged. Shoulders back; head up; a high-energy, confident walk; arms and hands relaxed; racquet up following a critical mistake meant two things: (1) nonempowering feelings of helplessness, doubt, and fear would not contaminate the competitor's chemistry, and (2) the competitor could take full advantage of the between-point recovery opportunity and thereby temporarily break the cycle of stress.

Skillful acting in Stage 1 paved the way for recovery in the next stage.

SECOND STAGE: THE RELAXATION RESPONSE

Stage 2 typically lasts six to twenty seconds and is accompanied by declining heart rates, blood pressure, muscle tension, respiration rate, and brain activity (EEG).

THIRD AND FOURTH STAGES:
THE PREPARATION AND RITUAL RESPONSES

The last two stages in the between-point time are called the preparation stage and the ritual stage. Once competitors stabilize their physiologies and are properly recovered, they can think clearly about the next point and plan their strategy. Without proper recovery, however, the entire competitive process is jeopardized.

NO RECOVERY—NO WAVES—NO GROWTH

Without recovery, stress is all there is. Stress becomes linear, constant, unremitting. Linear stress eventually means overtraining, increasing weakness, and poor performance. In a real sense, recovery is the foundation of toughness. Figure 9.1 depicts the fundamental role of recovery in the toughening process.

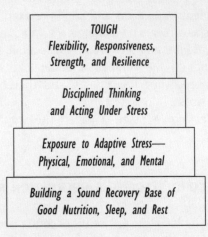

Figure 9.1 The Building Blocks of Toughness

It's important to understand that only rarely does the volume of stress defeat us; far more often the agent of defeat is insufficient capacity for recovery after the stress. Great stress simply requires great recovery. Your goal in toughness, therefore, is to be able to spike powerful waves of stress followed by equally powerful troughs of recovery. So here is an essential Toughness Training Principle:

WORK HARD.
RECOVER EQUALLY HARD.

From a training perspective then, training recovery should receive as much training attention as training stress. Unfortunately, this is rarely the case.

TRAINING THE MECHANISMS OF RECOVERY

For just a moment, let's review what recovery means. At the most basic level, recovery is simply anything that causes energy to be recaptured. Because the body expresses its recovery needs through feelings and emotions—for example, "I feel hungry," "I feel tired," "I feel lonely"—it's vital to respond to feelings.

In fact, the fulfillment of felt needs represents recovery. It's essential also to understand that recovery occurs in three areas— physical, mental, and emotional—just like stress. Recovery is also the period in which growth and healing occur.

The first step in training recovery is learning to recognize when recovery is occurring. In Chapter 7 I discussed the most common signs of physical recovery: reduced feelings of hunger, thirst, sleepiness, tension; slower heart and breath rates; decreasing blood pressure, muscle tension, and brain wave activity. The most common signs of emotional recovery are feelings of emotional relief; increased positive feelings of fun, joy, humor, and happiness; decreased negative feelings of anger, fear, and frustration; increased feelings of safety and security; and increased feelings of self-esteem, being loved, and personal fulfillment. The most common signs of mental recovery are feelings of mental relief; increased feelings of calmness; the sense of mentally slowing down; and increased feelings of fantasy, creativity, and imagery.

So now you know the signs of recovery. But how do you set out to actually *train* the mechanism of recovery? I've divided the training into the following five categories:

1. Sleep/naps
2. Diet
3. Active and passive rest
4. Seizing recovery opportunities
5. Emotional catharsis

SLEEP/NAPS

Along with food and water intake, sleep ranks highest in terms of recovery activities. Poor sleep habits can completely undermine the toughening process. Both too much sleep (excessive recovery) and not enough sleep (insufficient recovery) are problematic. Here are the most important Toughness Training Recommendations concerning sleep and naps:

- Get between eight and ten hours of sleep every night.
- Go to bed and get up within thirty minutes of your normal sleep times daily.
- Attempt to go to bed early and get up early whenever possible. Make every effort to reset your biological clock so that you become an early bird rather than a night owl.
- Learn to take short naps (ten to fifty minutes) and wake up feeling completely energized and refreshed. An afternoon nap as short as ten minutes can promote substantial recovery, particularly if it is synchronized to the body's natural urge to rest.
- Keep a daily record of the quantity and quality of your sleep, particularly during periods of high stress.

DIET

Consuming adequate amounts of water and nutritious food is a recovery activity of the highest priority. When nutritional and hydration needs are not met, all stress eventually becomes excessive and all other recovery mechanisms that are fundamental to growth fail. Here are the most important Toughness Training Recommendations concerning intake of food and water:

- Follow a consistent schedule of eating and drinking. This is a critical component of your overall training plan as an athlete.
- Always consume a nourishing breakfast.
- To stabilize weight, attempt to consume as many calories as you

are expending. Athletes may require more than 4,000 calories a day and up to 320 ounces of water during hot weather.

- Eat and drink every two hours whenever possible.
- Consume four to six meals per day, but eat lightly. Frequent small meals help to stabilize blood sugar, giving you more energy over longer periods.
- Whenever possible, eat early rather than late in the evening. Meals after eight-thirty are disruptive if you want to be asleep by ten-thirty or eleven.
- During endurance events lasting longer than one and a half hours, consume a liquid carbohydrate sport drink.
- Drink a minimum of eight glasses of water per day.
- Eat low-fat, carbohydrate-rich foods. At least sixty percent of your daily calories should be derived from carbohydrates, no more than twenty percent from fat, and ten to fifteen percent from protein.
- Eat as wide a variety of foods as possible, with a preference for natural, fresh foods that are free of preservatives and chemical contaminants. Eating a diversity of foods gives you the best chance of fulfilling all your nutritional needs.
- Avoid simple sugars, particularly around the time of competition. Simple sugars can spike blood sugar, resulting in a powerful release of insulin that may drive your blood sugar so far down you can't perform well.
- Consume carbohydrate-rich foods or drinks within two hours after an exhaustive workout or competition event. You have a window of approximately two hours to get optimal recovery benefit from the intake of carbohydrates. Replenishment of muscle glycogen stores is a critical recovery consideration.

NUTRITIONAL GUIDELINES

Consume more:

Fruits
Vegetables, particularly green leafy ones
Salads, pasta, rice, whole-grain breads, oatmeal, cereals that have
no sugar added
Egg whites, plain yogurt, turkey, and chicken
Meats and vegetables that have been broiled or grilled
Fruit juices and water

Consume less:

Fried meat
Red meat, no matter how it is cooked
Fried vegetables
Butter, margarine, mayonnaise
Creamy salad dressings: ranch, French, blue cheese, Thousand Is-
land, creamy Italian
Egg yolks, ice cream, doughnuts, pastries, cookies, candy

Consume fewer soft drinks and alcoholic beverages.

—————————————— **ACTIVE AND PASSIVE REST** ——————————————

The distinction between *active* and *passive* rest is based on the fact
that recovery from stress can occur both from movement and
nonmovement of the physical body.

Active rest involves nonvigorous physical activities that break
cycles of physical, emotional, and mental stress. Active rest for a
tennis player might be playing golf or playing catch with a Frisbee.
For a swimmer or diver it might be recreational biking, tennis, or
light jogging. Any activity that involves movement of the body and
breaks cycles of mental, physical, or emotional stress represents a
form of active rest. Other examples include the following:

- Walking
- Yoga
- Stretching
- Tai chi
- Fishing
- Noncompetitive, nonvigorous swimming, hiking, softball

Passive rest activities break cycles of stress without involving body movement. Watching a beautiful sunset, listening to your favorite music, and going for a relaxing drive are forms of passive rest. Other examples:

- Laughing
- Meditating
- Watching TV or a movie
- Getting a massage
- Reading
- Deep breathing
- Taking an afternoon nap
- Having a whirlpool bath

All of these, if done specifically to enhance the recovery process, are forms of recovery training.

SEIZING RECOVERY OPPORTUNITIES

All sports have built-in work/rest ratios. The work/rest ratio in tennis is approximately 1 to 2: ten seconds of stress during the point to twenty seconds of rest between points. On the other hand, golf has a very long ratio of rest to work, generally higher than 1 to 20 since over ninety-five percent of a round of golf's total time is spent between shots. Even the punishing game of football offers many recovery opportunities: huddles, time-outs, halftime, being benched, and so on.

An important aspect of recovery training is working to improve your ability to extract the maximum value from the recovery opportunities that exist during competitive play in your sport. Tennis players who practice their between-point walking, breathing, thinking patterns, and rituals are training recovery. Planning strategies for eating and drinking during competitive play also falls into the recovery category of training. Poor competitors invariably fail to take full advantage of the recovery opportunities that naturally exist in their sport. They also fail to see how training recovery mechanisms during play relate to competitive success.

Planning to better use your down time between competitive events and between practices is also very important in the context of recovery training. How you spend your time and with whom— when you're not competing or practicing—can make all the differences in the world in terms of how well you manage periods of intense competitive stress. Being certain you have your cassette player and favorite music tapes with you on trips, learning to sleep on airplanes and buses, and preparing nutritious snacks for travel days can make a significant contribution to your effort to achieve maximum performance at the most important times. The message is simply this:

$$CARPE \quad DIEM—$$

$$SEIZE \quad THE \quad DAY!$$

Seize recovery whenever and wherever the opportunity exists during periods of high stress. Here, as with so many aspects of competitive success, forethought and preparation make all the difference.

EMOTIONAL CATHARSIS

Two of the most powerful ways of achieving emotional recovery from disappointments, failures, and missed opportunities are through talking and writing about your feelings. Completely blocking the pain or denying your Real Self feelings prevents full recovery and perpetuates the cycle of emotional stress.

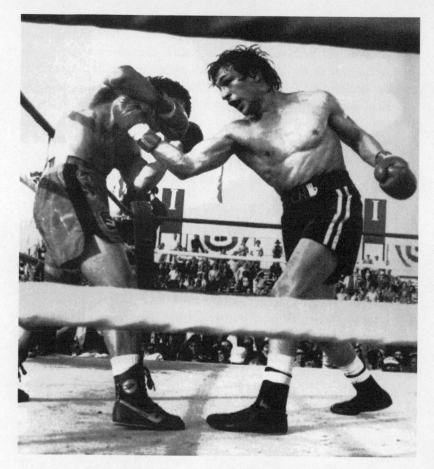

Ray "Boom-Boom" Mancini had the heart of a lion. The intensity of his training was greater than anything I had ever witnessed in my work with athletes. Ray used a library of humor tapes to help balance the stress of training. Twenty to thirty minutes of laughter daily helped to break the cycle of stress and increased his capacity for deep sleep.

The more you get into the habit of blocking your real feelings and emotions from expression, the less emotional flexibility and resiliency you will generally show in future stressful situations. Remember, negative feelings and emotions are generally blocked by the Performer Self during competition, but meeting the needs of the Real Self should clearly dominate during nonperformance times.

STRESS is the stimulus for growth.

RECOVERY is when you grow.

SUMMARY

Administering doses of stress and administering doses of recovery should receive equivalent training attention. Understanding the importance of recovery in achieving competitive success is essential. Learning to recognize how physical, mental, and emotional recovery feels—and how to fully use the recovery opportunities that exist both during and between competitions—is what recovery training is all about.

A vital realization is that insufficient capacity for recovery after the stress of competition defeats us more often than the volume of stress itself. In other words, frequently your ability to recover—physically, mentally, and emotionally—determines whether you win or lose.

As athletes we often fail to heed our body's cries for recovery. We also fail to recognize that opportunities for recovery exist everywhere.

To become stronger and to toughen, you must train daily to increase your capacity for, and understanding of, recovery.

10

THE IMPORTANCE OF

GETTING YOUR

REAL NEEDS MET

Feelings and emotions are the language of the Real Self and represent the principal vehicle through which the body gets its needs met—mentally, physically, and emotionally. And the body is constantly talking. To block feelings is to block the principal feedback mechanism that allows us to balance stress and recovery.

The Real Self simply can't power the Performer Self into its Ideal Performance State unless its real needs have been adequately met. At the extremes of deprivation, even mediocre performance is beyond reach. Imagine a well-trained marathon runner coming to the starting line after several days of fasting. Regardless of his level of mental toughness, not only has he sacrificed his opportunity to win, there's little chance he'll even finish the race.

Unmet needs on a much smaller scale can seriously affect performance potential: thirst, hunger, blood sugar imbalance, or lack of sleep—alone or in combination—can put the IPS beyond reach.

Unmet emotional needs can be equally disruptive. In this chapter the following questions will be addressed:

1. Which forms of need fulfillment are most important for athletes?
2. How is recovery related to need fulfillment?
3. Why is always being positive not recommended?
4. What is the meaning of negative arousal and how should athletes respond to negative feelings?
5. If athletes block out their real feelings through tough acting and tough thinking how can they get their needs met?
6. How can athletes separate important from unimportant needs?

The best way to answer these and related questions is to break the information down into specific principles. Let's begin.

PRINCIPLE #1: THE MOST NATURAL STATE IS POSITIVE

Positive emotional states are the norm for athletes when their needs are being adequately met; negative feelings and emotions signal unmet needs of some kind. Positive feelings therefore typically indicate stress/recovery balance; negative feelings indicate imbalance.

Healthy, balanced athletes find that their most normal state is positive and have discovered that they function best when their needs are registered against a positive state of mind.

Athletes who are always positive can't get their needs met because they never allow negative feelings to surface.

PRINCIPLE #2: EMOTIONS ARE THE EYES AND EARS OF THE BODY

The chemicals of emotion are messengers. They represent the internal instrument gauges for the body. Emotions are really flight data from mission control and, if properly interpreted, will faithfully guide you through life as well as through your performances.

Athletes who are blind to emotion remain chemically imbalanced and repeatedly fail to fulfill their performance potential.

PRINCIPLE #3: DECODING THE MESSAGES BEHIND EMOTION IS A MUST-LEARN SKILL

Often this is difficult because on the surface, feelings and emotions can appear bizarre, irrational, and unintelligible. Difficult as it may be, learning to decode the messages of emotion is the basis of self-understanding. Healthy athletes are those who have learned to get through all the cloud cover, who have learned how to trace negatives back to their source. Only then can they respond in ways that will fulfill their unmet needs. Tracing feelings to their source is like detective work. Sometimes the answer is obvious, but at other times a great deal of digging and investigation is necessary to get the right answer.

PRINCIPLE #4: NEED FULFILLMENT BRINGS RECOVERY

As you have learned in previous chapters, unfulfilled needs represent stress; fulfillment of needs represents recovery. Nontough athletes are those who repeatedly fail to meet important needs, and therefore suffer from the constant stress of chronic overtraining. Chronic stress invariably leads to chronic negativism, an emotional state that multiplies the difficulties of the decoding process. Understanding the needs behind chronic negativism can be mind-boggling.

Nontough athletes constantly find themselves doing things that bring temporary relief but do not meet the original needs. The use of alcohol and drugs to relieve emotional stress, or binge eating to relieve needs for love and affection, are examples.

PRINCIPLE #5: LEARNING TO LISTEN
AND RESPOND BRINGS BALANCE

Healthy, tough athletes are those who know what their real needs are and respond in ways that meet those needs as directly as possible. Negative feelings and emotions are allowed to surface against a predominantly positive mental state and traced as directly as possible to the source. For example:

"I'm feeling tired and irritated—my blood sugar is probably low. I'll eat something and take a fifteen-minute break."
"I'm feeling angry and upset, probably because my self-esteem is shaky. What I really need is more respect and attention from my coach. I'll schedule an appointment with the coach and talk about it."

PRINCIPLE #6: NEGATIVE EMOTION SERVES A PURPOSE

Blind suppression of negative emotion virtually guarantees that needs will remain unmet. A good analogy is that of a ringing phone. A need of some kind builds until it finally breaks through into awareness, much as a ringing phone finally gets your attention. The phone ringing represents the negative feeling. Most needs get progressively harder to ignore until you finally answer the phone and meet the need. Hunger is a good example. If you answer the phone and respond accordingly, the ringing stops. As long as you fail to eat, the phone will continue to ring—getting harder and harder to ignore. Eventually the ring becomes so distracting that either you disconnect the phone or you meet the need.

Disconnecting from negative feelings is not unlike covering the instrument gauges on a high-performance race car. You have no way of monitoring how things are really going.

Nontough athletes respond to negative emotion in the following ways:

1. They deny it altogether and remain eternally positive. They simply disconnect their phone lines.

2. They freely express whatever negative emotion happens to surface at the time, regardless of the circumstances. They hear the phone ringing and outwardly express their unhappiness with the nagging ring.

3. They'll do anything they can to get temporary relief from the phone ringing. Alcohol, drugs, and empty promises are examples. Temporarily shutting down the ring brings relief, but means the Real Self needs remain unmet—it's just a matter of time before the phone starts ringing again. Chronic negativism is the consequence of a consistent pattern of not meeting needs promptly and effectively.

Tough athletes respond to negative emotion in the following ways:

1. They hear the ring and answer the phone before it gets too distracting. Answering the phone simply means allowing the negative emotion to break into awareness so that the message can be taken. Some of these messages might be:

"I'm hungry—I need to eat."
"I'm tired—I need more sleep."
"I'm very nervous—I need to slow down and relax."
"I'm frustrated—my self-esteem is getting kicked around."

2. They decide whether the need being expressed is important or unimportant, rational or irrational. Is this a life-threatening emergency, or is it really an insignificant and small-time need?

3. They answer the following two questions:

Is this the time and place to meet this need?
Is there anything constructive I can do right now to get relief?

If they're in the middle of a competitive event and can't do anything immediately, this is when they reactivate their tough thinking and tough acting skills. Every effort is made to suppress the negative emotion and access positive empowering emotions. What the tough athlete eventually does is hear the phone, answer it, and take the message if nothing can be done immediately. A promise is made to attend to the need as soon as possible.

PRINCIPLE #7: SEPARATING NEEDS FROM WANTS IS ESSENTIAL

Unlocking your potential as an athlete is directly linked to fulfillment of *basic needs,* not *wants.* You may want to stay out late but need to rest; you may want to eat junk food but need better nutrition; you may want to give up but need to keep fighting to improve your toughness; you may want to take the day off but need to train even harder; you may want to throw your racquet over the fence or wrap your golf club around a tree but need to improve your performer skills. It's easy to mistake wants for needs.

Parents who constantly fill their children's *wants* produce spoiled, weak children. Parents who constantly fill their children's basic needs produce strong, resilient children. Whining, complaining, and frustration resulting from unmet *wants* perpetuate the weakness.

Ask yourself: Does this emotional pain I'm feeling stem from *wants* or *needs?*

If your answer is *wants,* take a closer look. Is there a deeper need that should be explored? This represents an important step in self-discovery and self-understanding. Controlling *wants* brings discipline; meeting *needs* brings balance.

PRINCIPLE #8: NEEDS EXIST IN A HIERARCHY

Some needs clearly are more important than others. The psychologist Abraham Maslow asserted that needs function according to a highly specific hierarchy. Needs for food, water, and safety—referred to as deficiency needs—are more urgent and have a higher priority than needs for love or self-esteem, referred to as growth needs.

Maslow contended that deficiency needs associated with life's basic urges—hunger, thirst, sleep, safety—must be met before the higher-order growth needs can be satisfied. In the context of Toughness Training this means that failure to meet basic physical needs blocks recovery, not only for those needs but also for many needs higher in the hierarchy.

Unmet needs associated with poor nutrition, inadequate sleep, and poor hydration create powerful cycles of stress. The fastest road to overtraining is failure to adequately meet basic deficiency needs.

As seen in Figure 10.1, the most basic essential human need, according to the Toughness Training Model, is to expend and recover energy—that is, to make waves. The most important forms of stress involve movement and stimulation of the body; the most important forms of recovery involve proper eating, drinking, sleeping, and resting.

The essential point is:

ACHIEVING STRESS/RECOVERY BALANCE
IN SPORT REQUIRES THAT
BASIC PHYSICAL NEEDS BE
FAITHFULLY MET EVERY DAY.

Remember, no balance, *no sustained toughness.*

Also remember: "Fatigue makes cowards of us all!"

Clearly one of the single most important things you can do to prepare yourself for competition is to enter the battle fully recovered physically.

Figure 10.1 The Hierarchy of Recovery Needs

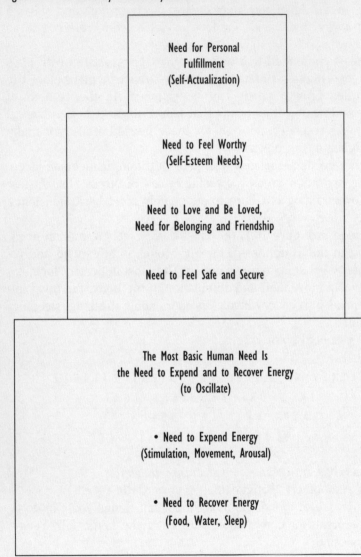

Adapted from Abraham Maslow's *Hierarchy of Needs,* 1962.

PRINCIPLE #9: CHOKING IN SPORT STEMS
FROM THE NEED FOR PSYCHOLOGICAL SAFETY

Fear of failure, of not meeting expectations, of looking bad can be as powerful and intense as fear of getting hurt physically. The more threatening a competitive event is to your psychological safety, the more stressful and disruptive it will be. Needs for psychological safety must be met or the hormones associated with fear will start creating havoc.

Fear simply signals increased stress. How you think and act *before, during,* and *after* competition greatly affects how threatening and disruptive the event is likely to be.

PRINCIPLE #10: SUPPRESSION OF NEEDS DURING
COMPETITION GENERALLY ENHANCES PERFORMANCE

Competition represents a major dose of stress. Feelings of fatigue, frustration, helplessness, anger, and fear are often stimulated. Tough acting and tough thinking are designed to move you away from disempowering (negative) feelings and toward empowering (positive) ones during competition. Acting as if you're not tired and not allowing yourself to think tired thoughts, however, suppresses need fulfillment. Your objective is to do the following:

1. Become aware of the need.
2. If nothing can be done to meet the need immediately, take the message.
3. Return to an empowered emotional state (suppress the negative emotion).
4. If the need is important, get relief as soon as possible after the competitive event.

SUMMARY

Listening to the messages the body sends via feelings and emotions is the only way we have of meeting essential needs. Unmet needs create powerful cycles of linear stress. Linear stress leads to over-training and a complete reversal of the toughening process.

The golden rule: *Remain sensitive to your body, to feelings and emotions, but never allow the chemical messengers of emotion to take control.* During competition you cannot be at the mercy of disem-powering emotions.

Make the commitment to meet important needs as soon as hu-manly possible, but as long as the battle rages, keep pushing your chemistry as close as you can toward your IPS. But if real pain is signaled at any time—in competition or not—give your undivided attention to the crisis.

TOUGHNESS TRAINING ASSIGNMENT

For the next two-week period, pay special attention to the fre-quency and meaning of the negative emotions you feel, both in and out of sport. Try to understand the source of unmet needs behind the negative feelings, the urgency and importance of those needs, and what you can do to meet any important Real Self needs as con-structively and directly as possible.

Gradually begin improving your abilities to understand your negative feelings and emotions, to differentiate between wants and needs, to meet important needs quickly and directly, and to sup-press the blow of critical negative emotion during competition.

11

THE ROLE

OF AWARENESS

Personal growth and positive change represent a lifelong pursuit both in and out of sport. This chapter focuses on a very simple but fundamental understanding:

PERSONAL AWARENESS IS THE FIRST
AND MOST IMPORTANT STEP IN
THE GROWTH AND CHANGE PROCESS.

In Chapter 4, you were asked to rate yourself on twenty-six personal factors related to competitive success. Your assignment was to confront the truth about yourself, to peel back the layers of protection and take an honest look at what's there.

Personal truth can be very scary. That's precisely why we build such elaborate defense systems—denial, repression, rationalization, and on and on. We simply want to protect our self-esteem from hurt; we desperately want to avoid pain.

As very young children we begin learning that one way to avoid emotional pain is to stop thinking about whatever bothers us. We learn that by pretending something didn't happen—or by blocking painful happenings from awareness—we simply don't hurt as much. Things are not as scary, as sad, as lonely, as disappointing, or as threatening. Blocking awareness can become a powerful strategy for reducing emotional pain. And the more painful the emotion, the more potential it has to block personal awareness.

Although it is somewhat effective in reducing pain, the problem with blunting personal awareness is that you progressively lose contact with the truth. In the context of the Toughness Training Model, the Real Self gets lost. The Performer Self grabs the reins and becomes whatever is necessary to keep from hurting—not just in competition but all the time.

Eventually the habitual pretending can become the dominant style of interaction. Unfortunately, when this happens, important needs associated with the Real Self go unmet. There's simply too much distortion. The instrument gauges that feed back critical stress/recovery messages no longer reflect what's really happening. Feelings and emotions can no longer be trusted.

And since stress/recovery balance is fundamental to the toughening process, the dimming of personal awareness eventually shuts the whole process down.

ATHLETES LACKING SELF-AWARENESS

Ungrounded, disconnected, and unresponsive are just a few of the words people use to describe athletes who lack good self-awareness. As a result, their greatest deficiency is poor self-understanding. Bill is a good example.

Bill, a seventeen-year-old tennis player, was referred to me by his mother and stepfather because, according to them and his coach, he consistently performed far below his potential. His coach described him as being unfocused and out of it most of the time. Bill has a long history of injuries. He presented a very superficial, almost phony image. He denied having any problems with nerves, pressure, or tension. He attributed most of his performance problems to bad luck and past injuries. The lowest score he gave himself on the CAP was a 6 on the patient-impatient scale. Most of his responses were 8s and 9s.

Bill was further described by his coach as defensive, undisciplined, and immature. The coach attributed most, if not all, of Bill's injuries to "stupidity" and sloppy training habits. "He just doesn't seem to learn from his mistakes ... he's always doing stupid things ... he forgets his keys, racquets, warm-ups ... he's on another planet most of the time."

From my perspective, Bill's most debilitating weaknesses were those emanating from his complete lack of self-awareness, self-understanding, and self-insight.

Bill eventually came to understand that his low self-awareness was his way of protecting himself from two very painful failures that had occurred much earlier in his life, neither of which were related to sport.

Fulfillment of Bill's athletic potential couldn't happen until he acquired significant insights regarding his Real Self. Over a period of several months, he made important breakthroughs and went on to become a successful collegiate player. The key factor in accelerating his personal growth was reawakening his self-awareness and directing it toward the goal of improved self-understanding. Bill showed considerable courage in his search for personal truth. Eventually the phoniness, forgetfulness, and defensiveness were replaced with a sense of realism and openness.

THE OPENING OF AWARENESS

Toughness and awareness seem like strange bedfellows, don't they? Yet for most of us, the journey toward toughness must follow the road of improved self-awareness and self-understanding. The deepening of personal awareness means becoming more open, more tuned in to the messages our bodies constantly send. It means listening and hearing the needs of our Real Selves.

Bill's assignment for several months remained essentially the same. He was to tune in and listen to his feelings and emotions, and to resist tuning out and hiding behind his protective mask of low self-awareness. He was to be particularly sensitive to any signs of defensiveness or insecurity. Each day he was to chart the following course with himself:

Step 1.   Increase his sense of self-awareness on a daily basis. *Where am I? What's happening now? What am I feeling?* Listen to the language of his body. Listen to the needs of his Real Self. Become aware when he started to hide and protect himself.

Step 2.   Pay special attention to negative feelings and emotions, particularly those of defensiveness and insecurity.

Step 3.   When he became aware of negative feelings he was to ask himself what needs were being expressed, and attempt to trace any hurt to its source. He was to try to understand and face his weaknesses—whenever he found them.

Step 4.   At the end of each day Bill was to evaluate his success with Steps 1 through 3. He was instructed to keep a diary, which I reviewed regularly. He was encouraged to express his *real* feelings and emotions for that day as openly and honestly as possible. He was also encouraged to be as courageous as possible in his search for personal truth.

Bill quickly realized that this four-step process is not an easy task. Some days were better than others, but every day was a struggle to some extent. Opening up to himself and the world was both threatening and confusing.

Bill's fear and doubt were gradually replaced with confidence, self-acceptance, and self-understanding. Bill has also come to understand that his daily four-step journey will never end. If he is to enjoy continued happiness, personal growth, and fulfillment, his search for personal truth and honesty can never end.

LEVELS OF AWARENESS

Understanding how levels of awareness relate to various states of consciousness can help shed important light on the toughening process. The highest level of awareness often is referred to as *conscious awareness.* It is one step beyond simple awareness. Awareness of your breathing, your pain, your joy, is one level of awareness, but awareness that you are aware of these things is quite another. The capacity to be aware that you are aware may in fact be one of the most distinctive features separating human beings from subhuman species.

The highest level of awareness is precisely what is necessary to accelerate personal change, growth, and toughening. Conscious awareness is self-reflective. It is through this self-observational process that new insights and new self-directions can be taken.

Bill's case is a good example. His deliberate effort to increase his personal awareness led him to a state of conscious awareness. To maximally accelerate the change process, he had to be more than just aware. Only through *a heightened state of personal awareness* could he consciously confront his weaknesses, consciously face them head-on, and vigilantly work toward the discovery of personal growth.

Once Bill began to learn new habits in self-awareness, once he began to tune in to the needs of his Real Self more automatically, the need for sustained conscious awareness steadily declined. His ordinary state of personal awareness had vastly improved. The fog surrounding his instrument gauges had substantially lifted.

Bill's accelerated personal growth required the highest level of self-awareness, referred to as *Level I Awareness.* Consciously training himself to be more aware deepened his capacity for the *Level II Awareness* that is simply his normal state of everyday awareness.

There are two additional levels of awareness that need to be discussed in the context of Bill's situation. These include the subconscious, referred to as *Level III Awareness,* and the unconscious, referred to as *Level IV Awareness.*

Here is a brief overview of what each level represents and how each pertained to Bill's problems.

LEVEL I: CONSCIOUSLY CONSCIOUS

This is the highest level of personal awareness. This is *being aware that you are aware.* Level I Awareness is the key to accelerating personal growth and toughening. Bill's assignment was to become consciously aware of Real Self needs, of old nonproductive habits, of weaknesses, and of new changes. Opening himself up to this type of awareness was both threatening and at times painful.

LEVEL II: CONSCIOUS

This is normal everyday awareness. Here you are simply aware of what's happening. Vast differences exist in Level II Awareness for most people. Bill began with little Level II Awareness, but made great improvement with training. Growth in Level II Awareness became possible only by diligently working with Level I Awareness.

LEVEL III: SUBCONSCIOUS

Here feelings, needs, and impulses remain just below your normal awareness. Bill's fog was the result of excessive subconscious functioning. Many of his needs and weaknesses remained just below his normal awareness. This learned pattern did serve to protect the Real Self from threat but prevented important needs from being met. Subconscious material is just outside of normal awareness but can be brought into awareness with conscious effort. Bill's increased self-understanding was the result of moving much of the material stored subconsciously into conscious awareness.

LEVEL IV: UNCONSCIOUS

This represents material that is essentially beyond the reach of normal awareness. Emotionally traumatic events can be stored by the brain so that they are not readily accessible to conscious awareness. This seems to occur instinctively to protect the body from what is perceived as a serious threat. Blocking traumatic events, preventing various thoughts, feelings, and emotions from entering awareness, acts essentially as a survival mechanism.

Blocking painful events from consciousness does provide short-term relief but often prevents healthy Real Self recovery. Depression, unhappiness, confusion, and low self-esteem can be traced to unconscious conflicts that have not been resolved. Many of Bill's problems stemmed from two such events that occurred early in his life. The first was the death of his father at the age of five, and the second was a near-fatal automobile accident that caused an agonizing four-week separation from his mother two years later. Only through talking, digging, writing, and conscious awareness did Bill finally get to the truth. His defensiveness, his playing stupid, his out-of-it way of relating to the world were now understandable.

SUMMARY

Becoming tougher, stronger, and more resilient requires an openness to change. That openness typically means expanding personal awareness to the highest possible level. Becoming *consciously aware* of your needs, your fears, and your personal weaknesses is the most critical step in the change process.

Self-understanding and the pursuit of personal truth require a keen sense of personal awareness. Blocking awareness brings temporary relief but eventually means the needs of the Real Self will not be heard. Balancing stress and recovery becomes impossible.

The healthy, balanced person is characterized by a clear sense of openness and nondefensiveness. Defensiveness always betrays weakness. Using conscious awareness to gain insight into your sub-conscious and unconscious worlds often results in great personal breakthroughs.

TOUGHNESS TRAINING ASSIGNMENT

For the next thirty days, you are to follow Bill's four-step program. Your goal is to increase self-awareness and self-understanding.

Step 1.   Increase your sense of self-awareness on a daily basis. *Where am I? What's happening now? What am I feeling?* Listen to the language of your body both during and between compe-titions. Listen to the needs of your Real Self. Become aware when you start to hide and protect yourself.

Step 2.   Pay special attention to negative feelings and emotions, par-ticularly those of defensiveness and insecurity.

Step 3.   When you become aware of negative feelings, ask yourself what needs are being expressed. Attempt to trace any hurt to its source. Try to understand and face your weaknesses—whenever you find them.

Step 4.   At the end of each day, evaluate your success with Steps 1 through 3. Keep a diary. Try to connect with your real feel-ings and emotions as openly and honestly as possible. Be courageous in your pursuit of personal truth. Once you dis-cover weakness or imbalance, take positive action immedi-ately.

12

TRAINING IN CYCLES:

UNDERSTANDING

PERIODIZATION

Periodization. It's a big word that may look a little overly scientific to many athletes. But every serious athlete should know and understand what it means. When you carefully follow periodization principles in your training, four things will happen:

1. You will reduce your risk of overtraining.
2. You will reduce your risk of undertraining.
3. You will reduce your risk of injuries.
4. You will increase the chances that you will perform at your peak when you want to most.

Let's tackle periodization head-on with a definition. Periodization is simply a long-term training plan that is designed to optimize your chances of performing at your peak when your most important competitive periods occur. Periodization really refers to wavemaking. To periodize means to alternate periods of stress with periods of recovery according to a carefully designed plan. The idea is that by properly balancing episodes of physical, mental, and emotional stress with episodes of physical, mental, and emotional recovery, the risk of injuries, staleness, burnout, and poor performance can be substantially reduced.

The concept of periodization was first introduced by a Soviet physiologist over twenty years ago. Much of Soviet and Eastern European success in international Olympic competition has been attributed to these athletes' understanding and application of periodization principles. Today periodization training has become the most accepted form of training among exercise physiologists and coaches worldwide.

WHAT ARE THE PERIODIZATION PRINCIPLES?

Periodization is an organized plan for implementing the following training principles:

- *Adaptation*
  This is the process your body goes through to get stronger, tougher, more resilient. The stimulus for adaptation is stress.
- *Frequency*
  This refers to how often the training stress should be applied. At this point in the year, should you increase or decrease the frequency of various training activities to meet your competitive goals? How many days in a row should you train and how many times per day is best?
- *Intensity*
  This refers to how hard the training stress should be applied. In other words, how hard should you be working at this point in your training program? How much weight should you be lifting, how fast should you be running, what percent of maximum effort should you be exerting?
- *Specificity*
  This refers to how similar the training stress should be to the

actual demands of competition. At this point in the year, how specific should your training be in terms of mirroring the actual stress of your sport? As a general rule, the closer you get to competitive events, the more specificity is called for in your training program.

■ *Variety*
This refers to how much variety should be used in the application of the training stress. At this point in the year, how important is it that you build change and variety into your training routines? Greater variety generally means more time for recovery and helps prevent staleness and boredom.

■ *Recovery*
This refers to how much time you should allow for adaptation and growth. At this point in the year, considering the frequency, intensity, and duration of your training, how much recovery time should be built into your program?

HOW TO APPLY PERIODIZATION PRINCIPLES TO YOUR SPORT

Some sports are seasonal, like basketball, football, and soccer; others have no defined season, like tennis and golf. Seasonal sports have built-in rest periods. Nonseasonal sports do not have defined competitive periods because competitive events typically occur year-round. Whether your sport is seasonal or nonseasonal, the principles of periodization can be of tremendous value in helping you achieve your competitive goals in the shortest possible time. Designing a yearlong periodization schedule focuses your attention on the big picture. Your periodization plan should help you provide solid answers to such questions as:

■ What are your most important competitive periods for the upcoming year?
■ When and how are you going to mobilize all of your resources so that you will have the best chance of peaking at the most important times?

- When and how will you specifically work to improve your cardiovascular as well as muscular endurance levels (improve aerobic capacity)?
- When during the year will you make any mechanical changes in your technique or form that might be limiting?
- When and how will you work to improve your muscle strength?
- When and how will you work to improve your speed and power?
- When and how will you improve your competitive skills (your Performer Self)?
- When and how will you schedule periods of rest and recovery?

Before you start building a periodization plan for your sport, you must understand:

- You cannot perform at peak levels all the time. A peaking cycle can be maintained for only about two to three weeks, and such cycles can only be achieved between three and five times within a given year.
- Every athlete is unique. The volume of stress you can handle, the volume of stress you must be exposed to in order to meet your needs, how much recovery you need, your ideal work/rest ratios for peaking are highly individual.
- The same careful planning should be invested in the scheduling and implementation of cycles of rest and recovery as in the scheduling and implementation of cycles of stress. In any periodization plan, stress and recovery should be given equivalent attention.

IMPLEMENTATION PLAN

Step 1:   List all your competitive events for the coming twelve months.
Include the dates and lengths of each competition. If your sport is seasonal, record seasonal dates, training camp dates, possible playoff dates. If your sport is year-round, list all events you intend to compete in, with dates and times.

Step 2:   Identify the year's most important competitive times for you.

Decide when the most critical peaking cycles will be during the next twelve-month period. What competitive events are most important? When do you need to be at your very best?

Step 3:   Pick your basic training cycle.

If you participate in sports having more than one season or play more than one seasonal sport, divide your year into a minimum of two six-month training cycles. If you participate in sports having only one well-defined season, use one twelve-month training cycle for your periodization plan.

Step 4:   Divide your six-month or twelve-month training cycles into the following training periods:

I.   Preparation Phase
II.   Basic Strength Phase
III. Speed-Power Phase
IV.   Peaking Phase
V.   Active Rest Phase

In each of these five phases, the principles of adaptation, frequency, intensity, specificity, variety, and recovery should be considered in your periodization plan.

Let's examine each one generally. Because of space limitations, this is only an introduction to periodization concepts. I highly recommend that you consult with experienced coaches, physical trainers, and sport psychologists who are familiar with your sport to help you design and implement your periodization plan. Every sport is different and requires a specific training plan.

PHASE I: PREPARATION

This is sometimes referred to as the aerobic or endurance phase. Your goal here is to develop cardiovascular and muscular endurance. Building a strong aerobic base is generally the first step in your periodization plan. Running, cycling, and cross-training with other sports are typically used during this time. Longer distances and slower repetitions for longer periods are emphasized. Thirty minutes of continuous activity within the aerobic training zone is considered minimal for most sports.

A complete break from all competition is called for in this phase. This is a good time to make mechanical changes in technique, form, and movement patterns.

Because competition has been suspended, the low emotional stress should promote an openness to new technical and tactical learning. This is an excellent time to review competitive goals for the season, to confront past physical and mental weaknesses, and to begin a process of rebuilding. Goal setting, self-analysis, and planning should be a central component of Phase I. This phase usually lasts two to four weeks.

PHASE II: BASIC STRENGTH

The focus of training here is on gaining strength in the movements and muscles specific to your sport: after this phase, you should realize significant gains in functional strength. Take care that this training component is designed and supervised by a competent professional.

Pay particular attention to areas of weakness and previous injury. Building strength is invariably the best insurance against injuries.

Although this basic strength phase refers to a specific physiological process, psychological considerations are also very important. Competition is generally not recommended during this period. Athletes should continue to work on their performer skills, rehearsing tough acting and tough thinking skills, listening carefully to the body's signals of overtraining, building solid self-talk habits, and so forth.

This phase lasts anywhere from three to several weeks.

PHASE III: SPEED POWER

Sometimes referred to as the precompetitive phase, this period is designed to develop explosive power and speed, particularly in sports where speed is especially important. For endurance sports such as cross-country running or distance swimming and sports such as golf and bowling, where explosive speed is not called for, the speed-power component is not emphasized.

Regardless of the sport, however, the specificity principle is very important here. Training should now mirror the actual physical and psychological demands of the sport as much as possible. Precompetitive routines, rituals, tough thinking, and tough acting skills should be fully engaged. Competition is highly encouraged during this period. The speed-power phase typically lasts two to four weeks.

PHASE IV: PEAKING

The objective here is to achieve maximum performance output in the context of competition. Power, strength, and speed are peaked by reducing the volume of training stress. Training sessions are generally of high intensity but short duration. The specificity principle is critical in this phase as well.

The days immediately preceding competition should be less demanding and less stressful both physically and emotionally. Your goal is to enter the peaking phase well recovered, rested, eager, enthusiastic, physically healthy, motivated, and confident. Competitive goals and rituals are of great importance during this time.

The peaking phase lasts anywhere from one to three weeks but can be extended by carefully and skillfully scheduling periods of competitive rest—for example, two weeks of competition followed by one week of rest.

The training focus of athletes during the competitive cycle should simply be to maintain current fitness levels. Careful attention should be given to issues of diet, sleep, naps, fun, relaxation, and recovery.

PHASE V: ACTIVE REST

This phase is designed to reduce the physical and psychological stress associated with your sport to the lowest possible level. A complete break from the sport is typically recommended. The theme for the active rest phase is recovery.

It is important to maintain minimal fitness levels during this time, and the best way to do that is through various forms of cross-training with other sports. For the best results, disengage physically and emotionally from your own sport. No playing. No practicing. No competition. This phase should last anywhere from two to four weeks.

SUMMARY

Training in cycles requires more planning, more discipline, and more thought than simply doing whatever comes to mind or seems logical at the time. Peaking your mind and body is no easy task and rarely occurs by accident at the times you need it most. Setting goals to peak or recover at certain times and then planning your training activities accordingly will likely mean better performances, fewer injuries, and greater emotional strength—at the most important times.

Most athletes and coaches find that designing and following a well-planned periodization program makes all the difference in the world in terms of forward progress.

TOUGHNESS TRAINING ASSIGNMENT

1. Develop a complete periodization plan in the next twelve-month period. Divide the year into one twelve-month period or two six-month periods on the following basis:

I. Preparation Phase (Aerobic)
II. Basic Strength Phase
III. Speed-Power Phase
IV. Peaking Phase
V. Active Rest Phase

2. Set specific training goals for each phase and keep a daily record of what you actually did compared to what you were supposed to do.
3. Get professional help in designing your plan. Consult with competent physical trainers for the first three phases; you may need additional help from coaches and sport psychologists for the last two. Always work closely with your coach.
4. Keep an accurate record of your competitive results, to be used to help evaluate the effectiveness of your periodization plan for the next year.

13

LEARN

FROM THE

MILITARY

Night drops like a curtain on the windswept sands of Iraq, where Operation Desert Storm is about to be unleashed. In a forward outpost PFC Curtis Lanateer, a nineteen-year-old American soldier, waits tensely for the order to advance into enemy territory. It will be his first experience of combat.

At the moment his only duty is to remain alert and watchful, ready to fight instantly should Iraqi infantry assault his company's position. As he sweeps the barren ground ahead through his night-vision scope, Lanateer reflects that barely a year ago he was still in high school. Thinking of the careless kid he was then, he smiles.

In the crowded year in the Army that followed high school, he gained more than proficiency with infantry weapons and great physical fitness. He gained an utter conviction that he will go forward when the order comes—forward into he knows not what except that it will be dangerous beyond anything he's ever experienced. Without dwelling on the possibility, Lanateer knows this could easily be his last night on earth.

Would the high school kid he was a year ago go forward into the hazardous night? The thought makes Lanateer chuckle; he knows the answer. Frightened out of his wits, the high school kid would cower in the bottom of the sandbagged trench Lanateer's squad occupies.

Briefly, Lanateer wonders about the change he's undergone. He wants to live as much as the high school kid, yet he knows he now possesses a hard courage to face death that the schoolboy never felt and could never have comprehended.

"Discipline did it," Lanateer thinks, "discipline, feeling strong and tough, knowing my weapons, along with lots of other things the military beat into me."

Lanateer's worst time—so far—came just before sunset when an Iraqi artillery shell screamed in and exploded a scant twenty yards away. The shelling continued for what seemed a very long time—actually less than ten minutes—until massive American counterfire silenced the Iraqi guns.

Then comparative quiet descended on the desert. As darkness came on, an occasional flare threw its garish light over the moonlike landscape. Now Lanateer can hear sporadic machine-gun fire somewhere off to the left. Are American soldiers like him being killed by that fire?

At last the order to advance comes. Without an instant's hesitation, Lanateer leaps up and runs forward in his assigned position on his squad leader's right, his weapon at the ready. Doing otherwise never occurs to him. Moments later, his squad goes to ground, engages in its first firefight, captures some prisoners, and moves forward again without sustaining any casualties.

The fear PFC Lanateer felt waiting to go into combat is exactly the same emotion athletes have before going into competition. The difference is in degree, not in kind: the competing athlete lays his or her professional career on the line; the fighting soldier lays his or her life on the line. In both situations, reaching over fear into effective performance demands mental and emotional toughness.

The necessary level of toughness can only be achieved *by training for it systematically.*

However you might feel about the military, you must admit the effectiveness of its toughening system. It can take *un*disciplined, *un*focused, *un*brave teenagers and within eight weeks transform most of them into soldiers tough enough to conquer the ultimate fear—the fear of death.

This physical and emotional conversion of fearful adolescents into courageous combat soldiers in so short a time is an astonishing feat, even given the fact that mankind has been perfecting military training methods for five thousand years. The art of enticing—or forcing—young men to risk their lives in warfare has been a primary concern of the older men who make wars for at least that long.

But could the military succeed so well so quickly without using highly skilled and deliberately obnoxious drill instructors to dish out large and carefully orchestrated doses of mental, emotional, and physical stress to recruits?

Absolutely not. Without obnoxious drill instructors the military not only would fail to produce reliable soldiers quickly, it wouldn't be able to produce them at all.

Given the age-old success of the military system, I reasoned that studying it would yield many important insights into the toughening process, and many tried and tested methods. That assumption proved true, although getting to the useful things required me to brush aside many useless aspects of military life.

WHY MARCH?

For thousands of years men marched into battle. Although they're now more likely to ride vehicles into the fighting zone, new recruits still spend many hours marching in formation. Why does the practice of marching remain so central to the making of a soldier?

It's interesting that battles haven't been fought on the march since the age of gunpowder began several hundred years ago. No one marches on modern battlefields—they run, hide, jump into fox-holes, or charge forward. Nobody stays alive very long marching in the face of the enemy. It's clear that in times past when soldiers still marched *into* battle, that's *not* what they did during battle. Marching is for *between* battles.

Clearly this regimented practice of walking in a particular way somehow breeds courage, confidence, and decisiveness during battle. Let's examine the practice more closely.

First of all, how do marching soldiers look on the outside? You never see any visible sign of weakness. If a soldier is tired you'll never know it unless he or she collapses. No visible fatigue, no sagging shoulders, no negativism, no fear. What you see is total focus, confidence, positive energy, and precision. Every movement is decisive and clean, nothing sloppy or lazy. Every breath is synchronized to exact movement.

Marching prepares soldiers for battle by giving them practice in being decisive, and in looking strong and confident regardless of how they feel. It trains discipline, sustained concentration, decisiveness, and poise, all essential elements in conquering fear.

THE MARCH OF CHAMPIONS

Why didn't I see it earlier? All great tennis champions have that same walk between points—between their battles—that marching soldiers display. Top tough competitors show the same focus, confidence, energy, and precision that soldiers do when they walk. No weakness, nothing sloppy, nothing but strength. Tennis champions walk the way soldiers march to bolster courage and control. I've come to refer to it as the *matador walk*.

Practice looking and acting the way you want to feel in your performance situations. Doing that pays off in terms of victory in combat for soldiers; it can pay off in terms of victory in competition for you.

THE ART OF SOLDIER-MAKING—OR ATHLETE-MAKING

The transition from fearful adolescent to fearless—or at least enormously more confident—warrior occurs in response to the following requirements:

1. A strict code of acting and behaving under stress. This includes:
   - A disciplined way of responding to stress.
   - A precise way of walking—head and shoulders erect, chin up.
   - Quick and decisive response to commands—no hesitation tolerated.

2. No visible sign allowed of weakness or negative emotion of any kind in response to stress. The expression of negative emotion is simply not permitted. No matter how you feel—this is the way you act!

3. Regular exposure to high levels of mental, emotional, and physical training stress to accelerate the toughening process. Obnoxious drill instructors—very tough individuals in the street sense of the word—provide all three kinds of stress.

4. Precise control and regulation of cycles of sleep, eating, drinking, and rest. The regimen includes:

   - Up early and to bed early (lights out—no choice).
   - Mandatory meals including breakfast—no choice about timing, few choices about foods.

5. A rigorous physical fitness program. This essential component of the toughening process involves two elements:

   - Aerobic and anaerobic training.
   - Strength training.

6. An enforced schedule of trained recovery. This includes:

- The regimen outlined in 4 above.
- Regularly scheduled R&R.
- Enforced cycles of stress followed by enforced cycles of recovery.

UNDESIRABLE FEATURES OF THE MILITARY TRAINING SYSTEM

1. *The stripping of personal identity* and its replacement by group identity (uniforms and short haircuts) are not appropriate to non-military life. Where this does happen—primarily in gangs and cults—it indicates seriously low levels of self-esteem.

2. *Military values, skills, and beliefs* have little application to civilian life. Many, though not all, of the military skills (for example, close-order drill and use of heavy weapons) have no value except in a military career.

3. *Blind adherence to authority* is rarely appropriate outside the military. Decisions in the military are made by next higher command, not by the individual. Successful competitors in the fast-paced world of sport must make their own decisions.

4. *The mental and emotional inflexibility and rigidity* often associated with the military mind would severely limit the careers of athletes who must cope with the subtleties and swift changes of civilian life.

5. *Acquired dislike of physical exercise* is a common result of the pain and boredom of basic training. Although this blind reaction robs some people of all desire to remain physically fit, many others find that military service sets a pattern of fitness that they maintain throughout their lives.

THE ROLE OF THE OBNOXIOUS DRILL INSTRUCTOR

If the brass hats had to take the obnoxious DI out of the military training mix, the generals would insist that they couldn't toughen the troops fast enough. The DI serves as a powerful mental and emotional stressor. Remember, no stress, no growth.

As long as the recruits fight the DI, as long as they get their feelings hurt, feel insulted, abused, afraid, and angry, they confirm that they are not yet tough enough. Only when they can remain calm, fearless, and unruffled by the DI's obnoxious treatment have the toughening adaptations taken place.

Experienced DI's get very skillful at detecting weakness in recruits, and their response is always the same—apply more stress, not less. Protecting weaker recruits from stress is the last thing an experienced DI would do. Accelerating the toughening process in the military always involves exposure to increased stress followed by enforced recovery.

One of the most important criteria for entry into elite training units such as the Rangers, Seals, and Green Berets is the capacity to manage high volumes of physical, mental, and emotional stress. The more elite the training corps, the greater the exposure to training stress.

It's most unfortunate in sport when coaches decide to become obnoxious DI's to hasten the toughening process. It is particularly tragic for young athletes. The screaming, yelling, threats, and punishment will lead to many accelerated adaptations, but at a very heavy price—the steady undermining of the player's natural love for the sport. Once that love is killed off, or even seriously injured, the game is over—maybe for a lifetime. DI coaches win lots of battles but always end up losing the war.

A note here for those athletes who must face misguided coaches who—for whatever reason—elect to assume the obnoxious DI role. If you're in this situation, without being aware of what's happening you suddenly awaken to the reality that your interest has died, your motivation is gone, your drive has vanished.

In such situations, Level I awareness is the most powerful tool you have to protect your passion and love for your sport. Never allow any coach to dampen your spirit. View the misguided coach as an opportunity to accelerate your toughness and use Level I awareness to prevent the coach's treatment of you from eroding your love for the game.

With Level I awareness you can rise above the threats, abuse, and ridicule. You can see the coach for what he or she really is and commit to not allowing your attitude or energy to turn negative because of him or her. This simply becomes an exceptional opportunity for you to get tougher.

SUMMARY

A major component of competitive success is controlling fear. That's precisely what military training is all about. However, in sport, it's fear of failure, of looking bad, of not meeting expectations. In the military, it's *fear of death*. When you choke in sport you'll likely lose the game; when you choke in battle you'll likely lose your life.

The emotional transformation that occurs in young recruits in the span of two to three months' training is remarkable. Understanding how the military trains new soldiers to control the greatest fear of all, fear of dying, throws light on many key aspects of the toughening process. In brief military programs, recruits are transformed from fearful to fearless, from scared to courageous.

The military training formula is simple but powerful: a strict code of acting under stress; no visible sign of weakness or negative emotion of any kind; exposure to mental, emotional, and physical training stress; precise control of recovery cycles; a rigorous physical fitness program; and recovery training opportunities.

Many aspects of military training don't apply to sport. Many elements of basic training, however, provide valuable insights into the toughening process for athletes. Becoming a courageous fighter, a fearless soldier in battle, is a key not only to battlefield success but to success in competitive sport as well.

TOUGHNESS TRAINING ASSIGNMENT

1. Practice looking like a soldier during tough times. Adhere to a strict code of acting both in practice and in competition. Visualize yourself toughing it out through difficult competitive situations by never showing weakness, helplessness, fear, or negative emotion.

2. Write out a brief Courage Statement that nails down your determination never to show weakness in practice or competition. Make your Courage Statement as vivid and emotional as possible, and take a moment to *feel it intensely* before every practice session or competitive event. No whining, no complaining, nothing negative—no matter how bad it gets.

3. Resolve never, never to surrender! Fight your best as long as there's a second on the clock or a point to be played.

14

GETTING

TOUGH

PHYSICALLY

You know the emotional script: get challenged; have fun; feel confident, energetic, and positive; and be determined in battle. You also know why the script reads that way—the chemistry behind these emotions brings your talent and skill to life.

You can learn to control these empowering emotions in essentially two ways. The first I call *outside-in* training; the second is *inside-out* training.

Outside-in is *physical toughening;* inside-out is *mental toughening*. This chapter will deal with outside-in training, meaning from outside the body inward toward the emotional chemistry. In Chapter 15 the focus will be on inside-out training. As you'll see in this chapter, physical toughening means three things:

1. Improving your physical fitness
2. Looking and acting tougher on the outside
3. Being well recovered physically before going into battle

Let's look at all three more closely.

IMPROVING YOUR PHYSICAL FITNESS

Whether the battle is intense or mild, competing in any arena—physical, mental, or emotional—requires energy. When the energy is gone, the fight is all but over.

Great coaches have always understood the connection between fitness and confidence, and between fitness and ability to hold up under pressure.

So have the military, the police force, and the FBI. Fitness is simply a measure of your capacity for energy expenditure, for accepting stress. The fitter you are as an athlete, the greater has been your exposure to physical stress. That means you can take physical hits and keep going. You won't buckle as soon as you are physically pushed.

Being more physically fit also means you'll have more energy to fight mental and emotional battles. Becoming physically stronger and more responsive deepens your belief in yourself as well. You become confident that you *can* go the distance; you simply refuse to surrender. You truly start believing that you can turn things around, that you can handle anything your opponent throws at you.

The following understanding is critical:

ONE OF THE MOST EFFECTIVE STRATEGIES
FOR IMPROVING IPS CONTROL
IS FOR ATHLETES TO EXPOSE THEMSELVES
TO INCREASED PHYSICAL STRESS.

When done properly, greater exposure to physical stress will always lead to greater emotional toughness. For some athletes, raising their fitness to a new level automatically leads to important psychological breakthroughs.

Based on my experience with athletes over many years, here are the physical fitness priorities I recommend to you.

PRIORITY #1: EXPOSE YOURSELF TO ABDOMINAL STRESS

This may come as quite a surprise, but your abdominals and obliques (the muscles on the side of your lower abdominals) represent the core of all strength. Weak abdominals and poor fitness go hand in hand. Problems with movement, low-back pain, poor posture, and faulty breathing can be linked to abdominal weakness. Weak abdominals predispose you to injury and undermine the entire physical toughening process.

Athletes should do a minimum of 200 curl-ups or modified sit-ups per day.

PRIORITY #2: EXPOSE YOURSELF TO HEART AND LUNG STRESS

How much cardiorespiratory stress you expose yourself to should be determined in the context of your overall periodization plan. The important thing is that your heart and lungs be sufficiently challenged to meet your physical, mental, and emotional energy needs for however long or hard the battle might be.

Can your fighting spirit endure? Can you recover energy fast enough? Is the energy there to drive your muscles, your concentration, and your emotions?

The ratio of aerobic to anaerobic training is determined by the specific demands of your sport. Obviously a distance runner requires an altogether different capacity than a quarterback in football, but both must have a minimal base. Increasing heart and lung fitness can be accomplished via any number of exercise routines using the large muscles of the upper and lower body. Examples are running, cycling, swimming, and using a stationary bicycle, stair-climber, or cross-country skiing machine.

PRIORITY #3: EXPOSE YOURSELF
TO OVERALL MUSCULAR STRESS

Again, depending on the specific demands of your sport and the training phase you are in relative to your total periodization plan, regularly overloading your muscles with stress to increase overall strength is a must. The ability to generate and resist force is a major component of toughness. Weight machines, free weights, flexible tubing, and many other types of resistance training equipment can be used to achieve greater total body strength. Consultation with an experienced physical trainer who has demonstrated success in your sport is highly recommended. The point here is that being physically stronger automatically translates into more IPS control.

PRIORITY #4: EXPOSE AREAS PRONE TO INJURY
TO PROGRESSIVELY INCREASING STRESS

Just as we break under pressure at our weakest points emotionally, the same thing happens to us physically. How many times have you been forced out of competition because the same weak ankle, knee, or shoulder let you down again? How much confidence can you have when the threat of your knee's or ankle's breaking down hangs over you?

When an athlete has a physical weakness that is prone to injury, the natural instinct is to protect it. Since the weaker knee can't take as much stress as the healthy one, the impulse is simply not to push the weakened knee as much.

That's precisely why the weak knee eventually always breaks down again. The key to rebuilding confidence in that knee or ankle always is the same two-step procedure:

1. Protect the injured limb, tendon, or joint from stress immediately following the breakdown.
2. Expose the injured area to progressively increasing stress as soon as the injury has stabilized.

Another tragic mistake made by athletes after serious injury or surgery is to stop doing their rehabilitation exercises as soon as the injured knee or ankle is as strong as the healthy one. The injured limb should be taken to a much higher level of fitness than the healthy one. That obviously means more exposure to stress.

PRIORITY #5: EXPOSE MUSCLES TO THE STRESS OF DAILY STRETCHING

Injuries can have a devastating effect on confidence. Muscle flexibility plays a critical role in any injury prevention program. The most important stretches are those for the low back and hips, Achilles tendons and calves, hamstrings and quads, groin, and shoulders. Consult a knowledgeable physical trainer to design a stretching program specific to your sport and bodily needs. Total stretching time is generally no more than ten minutes tagged on at the end of your normal workout.

LOOKING AND ACTING TOUGHER

Tougher physically also means better acting with the body. As you learned in Chapter 3, great competitors are great actors. Because the connection between the way you feel and the way you act is so powerful, I often refer to the following concept as the First Rule of Toughness. Here it is:

PROJECT ON THE OUTSIDE THE WAY
YOU WANT TO FEEL ON THE INSIDE.

It's so important to understand the communication process between emotions and the muscles of your body. When you're angry, sad, or fearful the muscles of your face, shoulders, arms, and legs become stimulated in emotion-specific ways. You immediately start looking the way you feel: angry, sad, or afraid.

Unless, of course, you're a great competitor and it's competition time. Great competitors have learned to reverse the stimulation process. To achieve this feat, which is essential to their competitive success, they use the same transmission channels that consistent losers use. However, rather than allowing their emotions to stimulate their muscles in the losing way, they use their muscles to stimulate the emotions they want to feel in the winning way. The key can be stated in just nine words:

THE LINK BETWEEN EMOTIONS AND MUSCLES RUNS BOTH WAYS.

Here are some critical truths that you, as an athlete seeking to improve your competitive success, should carve into your consciousness so deeply you'll never forget to apply them in every practice and every competition:

1. The way you walk, the way you carry your head and shoulders, and the expressions flowing across your face stimulate targeted IPS emotions. Simply moving your facial muscles from helplessness to fight, or from anger to fun, can be enough to give your blood chemistry a generous boost in those winning directions.

2. Acting *as if* you feel a particular way stimulates emotion-specific changes in your body.

3. What begins as a faked emotion can quickly lead to genuine emotion—particularly in skilled actors.

4. Acting *as if* is a trained response. As with all training, the more you do it in practice, the better you'll be at making it work in competition.

Developing a strict code for the way you act and look in competition gives you a powerful tool for controlling the feelings that

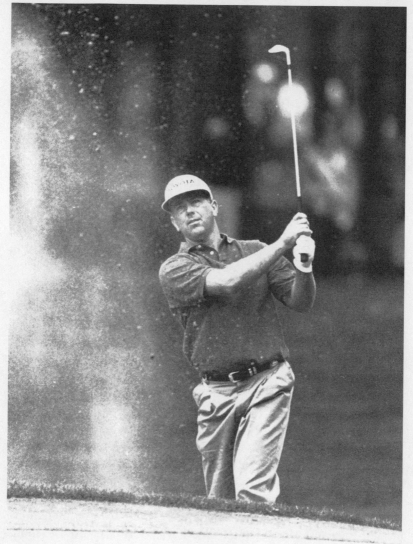

Great competitors have developed exceptional relaxation skills. No sign of tension of any kind is evident on Mark O'Meara's face as he blasts a pressure shot from the bunker. Mark's face is a picture of relaxed intensity.

lock out your talent and skill—feelings like fear, frustration, anger, and despair. Model yourself after the truly great ones like Michael Jordan and Wayne Gretzky. They're always sending the same messages with their bodies—calm, challenged, energetic, and confident. Remember, looking the way you feel enhances your current feeling. If you don't like your current emotional state, change the way you look.

BEING FULLY RECOVERED BEFORE BATTLE

The third arm of physical toughness is to enter battle fully recovered. The critical importance of recovery and of meeting the needs of your Real Self were presented in Chapters 7 through 10. The point I want to emphasize here is this:

> NO MATTER HOW TALENTED, SKILLED, PHYSICALLY FIT, OR MENTALLY TOUGH YOU ARE, IF YOU ARE NOT RECOVERED SUFFICIENTLY TO SUSTAIN THE ENERGY DEMANDS OF COMPETITION, IT'S OVER.

When glycogen (stored sugar) has been completely used up in your muscles, they can no longer properly contract and expend energy. When blood sugar falls below a certain point in your brain, precise concentration and clear thinking are not possible.

From my work with athletes for nearly twenty years, I have learned that many problems traditionally thought to be mental are, in fact, traceable to inadequate recovery. Here are three essential guidelines to follow:

1. Choose your recovery habits with care.
Undisciplined athletes who don't follow sensible rules regarding sleep, diet, and rest are the most likely to crack under pressure. In

other words, they collapse first. In the long run, undisciplined athletes always lose to disciplined athletes of the same ability.

2. Recover before your next competition.

Before taking on another dose of competitive stress, make every effort to be physically, mentally, and emotionally recovered. Most competitive events represent significant doses of competitive stress and therefore require considerable attention to issues of recovery.

3. Defend yourself against low blood sugar.

Guard against letting your blood sugar bottom out during or between competitive events. Remember to eat often and lightly. Complex carbohydrates in solid or liquid form will prevent low blood sugar from undermining your IPS. Be very careful not to consume simple carbohydrates like cookies, doughnuts, candy bars, and soft drinks before or during competition because they tend to spike blood sugar. A quick jolt of sugar causes the pancreas to release so much insulin that the body's blood sugar is driven down.

The necessity for a convenient between-meal snack is precisely why I urged our company to produce the Tough line of energy/recovery products: I believed there was a complete absence of convenient between-meal snacks for athletes that take up little space, can be easily and quickly consumed, have minimum spoilage problems, and don't create a lot of litter. Tough wafers and energy drink make it easier for athletes to stabilize blood sugar.

When properly used, sport drinks do the following:

1. Help meet daily carbohydrate intake requirements.
2. Help stabilize blood sugar.
3. Help restore muscle glycogen and liver glycogen.

SUMMARY

There is more to being a great competitor than merely being mentally tough. That's only half the battle. Being physically fit, possessing tough acting skills, and entering battle well recovered represent the other half of playing a winning game. It's vital for athletes to understand how everything is interconnected. Sleep, diet, fitness, free time, tough acting, and emotional toughness are all interrelated. Physical toughening, referred to as outside-in training, is an indispensable component of enduring competitive success.

TOUGHNESS TRAINING ASSIGNMENT

1. Develop a detailed physical fitness plan that is fully integrated into your periodization schedule for the year. Your plan should include concrete strategies for increasing abdominal strength, heart and lung capacity, and general overall muscle strength; for protecting against injury; and for improving flexibility. Consultation with a competent physical trainer is a must.

2. In every practice session constantly practice moving your chemistry in winning ways by improving your acting skills. Act the way you want to feel in practice so that you'll act in winning ways and move toward your IPS in competition.

3. Develop a detailed plan to ensure that you will enter battle fully recovered. Plan a schedule of meals, naps, sleep, snacks, and drinks that will meet your recovery goals.

15

GETTING

TOUGH

MENTALLY

Ideal Performance State control can be acquired in two ways. The first is by getting tougher physically through more outside-in training. Chapter 14 detailed how the control of empowering emotions can be accelerated through better fitness, better acting skills, and better recovery.

The second way IPS can be acquired is by getting tougher mentally. The connection between thoughts and emotions is very real. Getting tougher mentally means more inside-out training. It calls for learning when, how, and what to think and visualize before, during, and after competition to get the desired effect emotionally. Being tough mentally means that you have acquired skills in thinking, believing, and visualization that enable you to:

- Readily access empowering emotions during competition
- Quickly change from a negative emotional state to a positive one
- Cope emotionally with mistakes and failures

- Trigger an Ideal Performance State at will
- Cope with crisis and adversity

Mental toughness means that under the pressure of competition you can continue to think constructively, nondefensively, positively, and realistically—and do it with calm clarity.

STRATEGIES FOR GETTING TOUGHER MENTALLY

Helping athletes become stronger, more resilient, more flexible, and more responsive *mentally* has always been the greatest challenge in coaching. Both coaches and athletes have found the paths to better mechanics or better fitness far easier to follow than the path to training mental skills. My life's work has essentially been devoted to understanding and demystifying mental training for sport.

Here are my strategies for getting tougher mentally:

I. CHANGE YOUR THINKING TO CHANGE HOW YOU FEEL

The connection between thought and emotions works both ways: the way you're feeling affects the way you're thinking; the way you're thinking affects the way you're feeling. The important element here is that you can exercise substantial control over the direction and content of your thoughts.

That's precisely why great competitors are always disciplined thinkers. Sloppy, careless, negative thinking completely undermines IPS control.

Mentally tough athletes have learned to reverse the forces of negative emotion through tough thinking. As you learned in Chapter 3, tough thinking is simply thinking in ways that bring the emotions that empower you to life.

Overriding the temptation to think negatively because that's how you feel is no easy task. That's precisely why so many athletes fail to reach their full potential.

2. IF YOU DON'T LIKE THE FEELING, CHANGE THE PICTURE

Images are more powerful triggers of emotion than words. That's how actors and actresses are trained to perform emotionally. They are taught to skillfully use emotionally charged images to access the targeted emotions.

Tough competitors do the same thing. They consistently use images of success, of fighting back, of having fun, of staying relaxed, of being strong in the face of adversity, to move their chemistry in those directions.

However, if you expect to change fear into challenge, or disappointment into determined hope, practice is essential. The most powerful and important image you carry in your arsenal is your *self-image*. Work daily to make it strong, vivid, and courageous—and that's exactly what you'll get back in competition.

3. TAKE FULL RESPONSIBILITY FOR WHAT AND HOW YOU THINK

You've learned that negative feelings often serve the vital purpose of signaling important unmet needs of various kinds. You've also learned that negative feelings have no place in the Ideal Performance State. Do you go with the negative feelings and search for unmet needs, or do you block the negativism and go with IPS? The solution is fundamentally this:

MAKE EVERY EFFORT TO SUPPRESS
NEGATIVE FEELINGS DURING
COMPETITIVE BATTLE UNLESS
YOU CAN DO SOMETHING POSITIVE RIGHT
AWAY TO MEET THE EXPRESSED NEED.

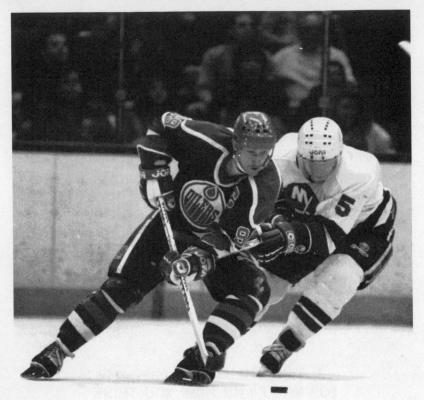

Wayne Gretzky attributes much of his success to his ability to set meaningful goals, to maintain a moment-to-moment focus during play, and to have fun as he performs.

One of the most powerful things you can do to suppress negative thoughts and feelings is to say "Stop" to yourself and immediately begin processing positive thoughts and images. Put your heart into not allowing negative feelings to lead you into negative thinking. *Negative thinking takes you nowhere competitively.*

You aren't always responsible for negative feelings, but you are always completely responsible for any negative thinking you permit. After all, nobody but you is inside your head.

— 4. CONSTANTLY PRACTICE POSITIVE THINKING —

Positive thinking and positive imagery skills are acquired in the same way motor skills are—through repetition. Sloppy, undisciplined motor movements lead to bad mechanical habits. The same principle holds true for sloppy, undisciplined thinking. Lazy, negative thinking in practice will come back to haunt you in competition the same way sloppy mechanics will. You've got to practice, practice, practice the right mental habits to be strong enough to hold up under the pressure and frustration of competition. That's exactly what being tough-minded means—you continue to think positively and constructively during the toughest of times.

— 5. NEVER THINK OR SAY CAN'T; — NEVER THINK OR SAY HATE

"I can't handle it. I can't stand it. I can't believe it. I can't do it. I can't make it ... I hate myself. I hate my opponent. I hate this place. I hate the coach. I hate mistakes." These are all examples of nontough thinking. They rapidly build emotional roadblocks. This type of inflexible, rigid thinking always leads to competitive problems.

— 6. THINK—VISUALIZE IN VIVID EMOTIONAL — TERMS—THESE THOUGHTS DAILY:

- "I will put myself on the line every day."
- "I will not surrender."
- "I will not turn against myself during tough times."
- "I will come totally prepared to compete every day."
- "I will not show weakness on the outside."
- "The crazier it gets, the more I will love it."
- "I love competing more than winning."

7. THINK HUMOROUSLY TO BREAK UP NEGATIVE EMOTIONS

When you think nutty, goofy, silly, funny, off-the-wall thoughts, fear and anger vaporize. When you are overly aroused with emotion, internal laughter puts you back in control. Use humor with teammates when you sense that arousal levels are getting too high. Think about things that break you up from the inside—things that make you start jiggling internally with laughter.

8. THINK MORE ENERGETICALLY

Energy is everything, and attaining a high level of *positive energy* is the key to competitive success. Get more positive emotion flowing during battle by thinking more energetically. Think "fun" and more positive energy will start flowing immediately. Think or say out loud:

"I love it!"
"Yes!"
"Is this great pressure or what?"

9. LEARN TO KEEP A HERE-AND-NOW FOCUS DURING COMPETITION

Here's one of the greatest secrets of peak performance in sport: sustaining a here-and-now mental focus during competition makes the natural expression of talent and skill far easier. A present-centered focus, particularly during critical moments of execution, is fundamental to performing well under pressure. *During battle, thinking about the future lets fear beat you; thinking about the past lets anger and frustration beat you.* Practice maintaining a moment-by-moment focus during practice and competition.

Use Level I awareness to accelerate the learning process (see Chapter 11).

— 10. DURING CRITICAL MOMENTS OF EXECUTION, — —— FOCUS YOUR ATTENTION OUTSIDE YOURSELF ——

Choking often occurs because too much attention is focused inward. Being aware is one thing—being self-conscious is quite another. The more you can get "outside your head" and completely absorbed in the activity itself, the better you will typically perform.

Focusing on a precise target just before critical execution brings a narrow, external concentration that enhances performance for most athletes. Again, considerable practice is needed to control attention when things get rough. Emotion and attention are powerfully connected.

Negative emotions lead to arousal problems and arousal problems lead to attention problems. Learning to direct your attention to the right targets and away from the wrong ones keeps negative emotions in check and helps you achieve proper arousal. Again, use Level I awareness and lots of practice to hone attention skills.

———————— 11. PRACTICE STRATEGIC ——————— ———————— VISUALIZATION CONSTANTLY ————————

"See," "hear," and "feel" yourself overcome your weaknesses and accomplish important goals. Experience victory and success *mentally* before you test yourself *physically*. Use mirrors, photographs, and video replay to strengthen and improve the accuracy of the mental pictures you have of yourself performing. Mentally rehearse difficult physical routines that have given you trouble, such as fielding, shooting, jumping, turning, or hitting. The physical practice of a skill accompanied by appropriate mental practice is far superior to physical practice alone.

Remember, visualization works best when you have achieved a deep state of calmness and relaxation (see Chapter 16). Many short sessions (five to ten minutes) are much better than one or two long sessions.

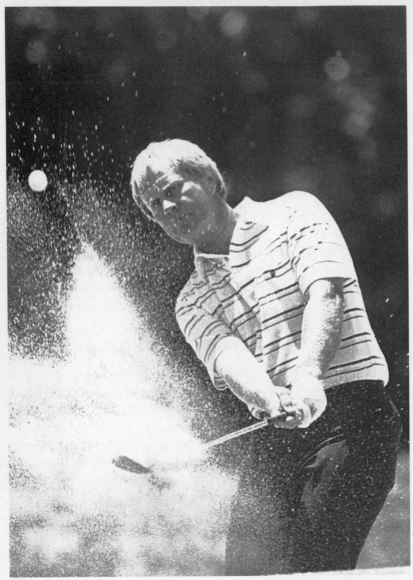

Jack Nicklaus is considered by many to be the greatest competitor golf has ever known. He attributes his toughness to two things—his ability to vividly visualize each shot before making it and his ability to create waves of relaxation between shots and waves of intense focus and concentration prior to and during shots. He was simply a better wave maker.

──── 12. BE MORE DISCIPLINED IN THE WAY ────
──── YOU THINK ABOUT YOUR MISTAKES ────

If you fear mistakes, you will make them. If you fear losing, you will lose. Playing not to lose or not to make mistakes locks you up inside and has tragic performance consequences. How you think about mistakes has a major impact on the emotional state you carry into battle. Here's the winning way to think about mistakes:

"Mistakes are a necessary part of learning. No mistakes—no learning. I'll make my mistakes fearlessly and aggressively. I'm not playing it safe, holding back or looking for excuses. I'm going for it—I'll accept whatever happens and move on. I don't fear mistakes; I learn from them."

After making a painful mistake, ask yourself these three questions and move on:

1. What could I or should I have done differently?
2. What can I learn from this?
3. What can I take away from this that will help me in the future?

Once these questions have been answered, make a conscious decision to let it go!

──── 13. BE CLEAR WHY IT'S IMPORTANT ────
──── TO FIGHT BEFORE THE BATTLE BEGINS; ────
──── THEN MAKE THE COMMITMENT ────

Without a clear commitment to fight, you probably won't. It's just too painful and requires too much energy. Why are you competing? Why are you here? How important is this contest for you? Are you willing to commit 100 percent emotionally to the battle? Will you put yourself totally on the line and risk losing—giving everything you have to give?

—— 14. USE ADVERSITY TO GET STRONGER ——

Just like mistakes, the way you think about adversity and crisis largely determines the impact these things will have on you. Every crisis is an opportunity to grow, to reach further, to extend beyond your normal limits. A major component of emotional toughness is learning the right attitudes regarding tough times. "Tough times are stress. Give me stress, it's the only way I'm going to get tougher."

—— 15. CONSTANTLY REMIND YOURSELF —— TO LOVE THE BATTLE ——

Love the process, the fight, the marshaling of your resources, the pushing, the falling back, the breakthroughs, the struggles. Loving to win is easy. Loving the process moves you to a whole new level of competitive skill. Loving the battle happens because you make it happen.

—— 16. USE POSITIVE BRAINWASHING —— TO BREAK NEGATIVE MENTAL HABITS ——

The world is constantly conditioning you to develop negative habits of thinking and acting. And the conditioning process is very powerful. That's why so many athletes have developed so many negative mental habits. Negative self-talk, negative thinking of all kinds: "I can't do this . . . I can't do that . . . I hate this . . . I hate that . . ." and on and on.

Use Level I awareness to identify the negative mental habits that hurt you in sport and start the process of *positive brainwashing*.

Let's assume you are a golfer, and over time you have developed some very negative attitudes about putting. Your thinking is essentially this: "I'm a lousy putter. I hate putting. I have no feel for putting. I'll never make it competitively because of my damn putting skills."

Positive brainwashing involves the following steps:

1. Make signs that read "I Love Putting" and put them everywhere. Put them on your refrigerator, your bathroom mirror, the dashboard of your car, so that everywhere you look you are reminded that you now *love putting*.

2. For the next thirty days, write "I Love Putting" twenty-five times a day. As you write the phrase, say it to yourself with conviction.

3. Every time you approach a green during play, say to yourself, "I love putting," and then break into a smile.

It will take between twenty and thirty days before new mental habits start taking form. Although the process seems rather silly, it is remarkably effective. You can use the same basic procedure for a wide variety of negative mental habits.

17. JUST FOR TODAY

Use the "just for today" approach to changing your habits. Here are some "just for today" resolutions to make to yourself.

"Just for today, I will become challenged when problems come my way. Today I will be a great problem-solver."

"Just for today, I will love the battle. I can create my own state of enjoyment. I will accept the hand that is dealt to me. No complaining!"

"Just for today, I will exercise, eat, and train right. Self-discipline will bring the confidence I search for."

"Just for today, I will take charge of how I feel. I am not at the mercy of my emotions."

"Just for today, I will set aside some time to relax and simply let go. Relaxation is an essential part of training."

"Just for today, I will have a plan to follow. The plan will keep me focused and organized."

"Just for today, I will stop saying, 'If I had time.' If I want time, I will take it."

"Just for today, I will find humor in my mistakes. When I can smile inside, I am in control."

"Just for today, I will do things the best I can. I will be satisfied with what I have done."

"Just for today, I will do the ordinary things in my training extraordinarily well. It's the little things that make the difference."

"Just for today, I will choose to believe that I can make the difference and that I am in control of my world."

"Just for today, *the choice is mine.*"

SUMMARY

Mental toughness plays a powerful role in Ideal Performance State control. It consists of acquired skills in positive thinking, humor, problem-solving, tough thinking, visualization, and tough believing. Mental toughness training is inside-out training that is designed to help athletes become mentally more flexible, responsive, strong, and resilient under pressure. This chapter presented seventeen training strategies to accelerate the mental toughening process:

1. Change your thinking to change the way you feel.
2. Change the picture if you don't like the feeling.

3. Take full responsibility for what and how you think.
4. Practice positive thinking constantly.
5. Never think or say "I can't"; never think or say "I hate."
6. Think empowering thoughts.
7. Think humorously to break up negative emotions.
8. Think more energetically.
9. Learn to keep a here-and-now focus during competition.
10. During critical moments of execution, focus your attention outside yourself.
11. Practice strategic visualization constantly.
12. Be more disciplined in the way you think about your mistakes.
13. Be clear why it's important to fight. Before the battle begins, make the commitment.
14. Use adversity to get stronger.
15. Constantly remind yourself to love the battle.
16. Use positive brainwashing to break negative mental habits.
17. Focus on "Just for today."

TOUGHNESS TRAINING ASSIGNMENT

From the seventeen strategies for getting tougher in this chapter, select the two that most directly address the weakest points in your mental toughness. Then start right now and put all the energy and determination you can command into making them work for you.

Once the first two strategies you select are up and running, choose the next two strategies that are most relevant to your needs. Continue until you have acquired all the necessary mental toughness skills.

For more detailed information about mental toughening strategies, I recommend that you read my book *Mental Toughness Training for Sports*. Athletes in a wide variety of sports have found it very helpful.

16

TRAINING

BRAIN

WAVES

Your brain makes waves constantly. The frequency and amplitude of the waves can be measured with an electroencephalogram (EEG recording device). Everything from concentration to fear and from imagery to relaxation is directly linked to brain wave activity.

Your Ideal Performance State is directly connected to a particular pattern of neurological (brain) arousal. In this chapter we will explore ways to improve concentration, visualization, and relaxation skills through an enhanced understanding of the way the brain works.

THE FUTURE

Imagine this. You're a highly ranked tennis player and your most important competitive event of the year comes up in three weeks. Today you begin your normal precompetitive mental training program. Thirty minutes per day for twenty-one days is all it takes. The program works like magic, protecting you from nerves and enabling you to perform to your best when you need it most. It's a little boring but well worth the effort.

You take a seat, lean over, and start flipping switches: computer link, microprocessor, and video display terminal. You put gel on the six electrode sites and settle the EEG cap over the top of your head. You punch two commands into the keyboard and suddenly the multicolored display terminal in front of you comes alive. You fidget with the EEG cap until all leads show hot on the computer screen, and zappo, there it is—your living, breathing brain staring at you straight on.

Right side, left side, four quadrants and colors—lots of colors. You begin with an EEG scan for baseline data. The high-frequency beta in both hemispheres comes as no surprise because you've been stressed out for two days after receiving bad news about your mother's health. Today is going to be very challenging. Considering how uptight and edgy you feel, achieving your IPS pattern for any length of time will be very tough, especially since you haven't practiced on the EEG training unit for nearly two months.

You begin. Continuous visual and auditory feedback tells you when your brain wave activity is moving toward—or away from—the desired IPS pattern. Information on beta, alpha, theta, and delta frequencies for both hemispheres flows continuously across the screen.

Frequencies between 14 and 40 cycles per second increase, and the beta channel comes alive, 8 to 13 for alpha, 4 to 7 for theta, and less than 4 for delta. With all the mental training you've done, you know exactly how each frequency band feels. High-range beta, particularly left side, is *stress*—you're edgy, uptight, defensive, angry, afraid. All the wrong stuff. Unfortunately that's where you are right now. Lots of beta everywhere. Alpha feels free, relaxed, easy, but still connected. Theta is out there—spacy, drifting, sleepy, floating, images far out. Delta is gonzo, history, sleepsville.

It took several staged competitive events using on-court telemetry to lock in on your IPS pattern, but the computer memory has got it now. Everybody is a little different, so canned IPS programs are not as effective. Yours is right on.

Nine minutes and fifteen seconds into the training program and you finally start homing in on the targeted frequencies. You're still not sure how or why your brain waves change when you decide to move them, but with the feedback they just start going in the right directions. After ten or more sessions you actually start getting pretty good.

Bingo. Eleven seconds flat. The monitor lights up and the tones start singing. The IPS light and sound show finally arrives. For you, IPS is just on the cusp of beta and alpha—12 to 14 cycles per second with synchrony. Your right and left hemispheres are perfectly balanced.

For the next ten minutes you struggle to keep IPS rolling. Today it's tough. Too much personal stress and not enough practice. But now that part I is out of the way you can cruise. Part II is a trip to your theta window. The only thing you have to worry about now is falling asleep.

You tell yourself, "Let go—drift, sleepy, slow float." Gradually your frequencies get slower and slower. When your eyes are closed, a tone finally signals theta. You're there. Now the programming begins—prerecorded messages start coming through the headphones in your own voice. "You love to fight. Competition is fun for you. You stay relaxed and calm in tough situations."

And the messages keep coming. All the things you need to hear at the most important time to hear them—in the theta window. You're not sure how or why it works—only that it does work. What you've come to understand is that whatever information is dumped into your brain while theta flows tends to stick. Problems with nerves, confidence, concentration, and negative thinking, can be targeted in theta. The whole process still amazes you.

The last seven minutes is spent mentally rehearsing the way you want to perform in your upcoming tournament. Repeated visualization practice during slow brain wave activity (alpha-theta) has clearly accelerated your competitive skills.

Thirty-one minutes and eleven seconds into your mental training session, you start flipping the off switches. You're out of there.

SCIENCE FICTION OR REALITY?

The scene just described is not fiction. It's actually happening today. So sophisticated is the technology that we can now accurately measure down to 1/100 of a microvolt. That's a millionth of a volt!

Since we can now detect a single neuron firing in the brain, it's clear that we've come a long way from the crude biofeedback equipment of the 1970s and 1980s.

This new era of brain wave training is called *EEG neurofeedback*. It's now being applied in a diversity of research areas that include:

- Helping children with attention problems, called *attention deficit hyperactivity disorders* or *ADHD*
- Helping individuals overcome the negative emotional effects of traumatic events such as rape or hurricanes, called *post-traumatic stress disorder*
- Helping Vietnam veterans overcome the emotional trauma of war, called *post-Vietnam syndrome*
- Helping rehabilitate individuals who have suffered severe head injuries, called *closed head trauma*

The work of Lubar, Everly, Keltner and others shows great promise for multiple applications of EEG neurofeedback technology. The most promising research has been conducted by Dr. Eugene Peniston in the treatment of alcoholism and drug addiction. His success rates in breaking addiction through accessing what he calls "the EEG window of opportunity" are unparalleled.

The application of EEG neurofeedback to athletic performance is still in round one, but preliminary results are most promising. Several researchers are intensively studying the specific neurological patterns that occur during periods of peak performance (zoning).

WHAT CAN YOU DO NOW?

Although the cost of such equipment is declining fast, most athletes will not have access to such technology for some time. But much can be done today without precise instrumentation. Based on years of study by a great number of excellent researchers in the areas of visualization, relaxation, concentration, and biofeedback; based on my own work and experience with athletes for nearly twenty years; and based on the new findings in EEG neurofeedback research, here are my recommendations for what you can do *now*.

PRACTICE SOME FORM OF RELAXATION TRAINING REGULARLY

Your goal is to learn how to slow down brain wave activity on command. Most concentration and competition problems stem from excessive neurological arousal (brain wave patterns are too fast). Pressure, nerves, fear, anger, and frustration serve to increase EEG frequency. Breath control training, meditation training, yoga, listening to specially prepared relaxation audiotapes, and progressive relaxation exercises can all be used for this purpose.

Progressive relaxation exercises have been very popular with athletes. This simply involves systematically tensing and relaxing specific muscle groups. Voluntary relaxation of muscles is paired with the cue to relax. Decreasing muscle tension is generally accompanied by decreasing brain wave frequency. EEG research clearly shows that the more you practice slowing down brain waves, the better you get at it.

——— PRACTICE VISUALIZATION TRAINING DAILY ———

Learn to picture things so vividly in your mind you can actually hear, see, feel, and touch them. This represents an absolutely essential performer skill that is clearly acquired with practice. Your brain is unable to differentiate something vividly imagined from actual reality. Great competitors are invariably great visualizers. They have learned to project themselves into the future and actually "see" themselves achieving important goals in their minds long before the actual event. Being prepared mentally and emotionally is nearly synonymous with visualization practice.

– FOR THE BEST RESULTS, PRACTICE VISUALIZATION – ——— WHEN YOU ARE DEEPLY RELAXED ———

If Eugene Peniston and others are correct about the theta window, self-suggestion and visualization will have the most profound effects if done during very slow brain wave frequencies. Most people describe the theta state as a dreamlike state that occurs just before sleep.

One explanation for why the assimilation of information may be so much more powerful during slow brain wave states is that the rational, logical filters have been suspended. Critical, logical, defensive thinking occurs when the dominant hemisphere is very active.

During relaxation your brain is more open and receptive to material that might normally be rejected. In normal, more rational states of consciousness, self-affirmations like "I am strong and confident" might be readily discarded because they are logically judged to be trivial, irrational, or untrue.

——— VISUALIZE YOURSELF OVERCOMING ——— ——— YOUR GREATEST WEAKNESSES ———

From fearful to fearless, weak to strong, defensive to open, negative to positive, impatient to patient, passive to aggressive—attack your mental weaknesses on many fronts, but most importantly crystallize the breakthroughs with real-life images—over and over.

If you need to be more aggressive and assertive under pressure, vividly imagine yourself being exactly that in competition. Create tough situations in your imagination and "see" yourself competing assertively to achieve your best performance. "Seeing" the changes become a reality in your imagination is a critical step in converting weakness into strength.

PLAY CAREFULLY PREPARED TAPED MESSAGES DURING PERIODS OF DEEP RELAXATION

Someday research may link the theta window to the mysterious phenomenon of hypnosis. Could it be that being hypnotized simply means accessing a particular brain wave frequency called theta? Are easily hypnotized individuals commonly those who have learned to easily produce high concentrations of theta waves? Logic certainly suggests a connection.

In any case, my experience with athletes—as well as the experience of many other sport psychologists—regarding the playing of audio messages during deep relaxation strongly confirms its potential value. Positive affirmations, positive suggestions, and positive images introduced during cycles of slow brain wave activity can accelerate the process of personal change in an exciting way.

Slow brain wave activity and theta frequencies in particular can provide access to subconscious and unconscious information that would ordinarily be unreachable. Flashes of great insight are not uncommon during deep relaxation. This is why theta and delta frequencies are now being referred to by some as *the healing frequencies*.

CONCENTRATE IN PRACTICE

In plain words, concentrating means paying attention to what's important and blocking out what's not. Researchers have found that children with attention problems are often stuck in alpha and theta frequencies without being able to produce sustained beta.

Clearly, intense concentration reflects highly specific states of neurological arousal. The more you practice homing in on the right frequencies, the more control over concentration you will develop. That's precisely why emotional states and concentration are so interconnected. Anger, fear, and frustration interfere with concentration because these emotions increase neurological arousal. Depression, sadness, and low motivation interfere for precisely the opposite reason. The emotional state consistently linked to successful concentration is one characterized by feelings of high positive energy, fun, and enjoyment. You rarely if ever need be reminded to concentrate when the state of fun has been established. Researchers will one day, no doubt, map the neurological differences between fun and nonfun emotional states.

The connection between concentration and neurological arousal certainly helps explain why relaxation training often leads to significant improvement in concentration skills during competition. The natural pressures of competition typically increase brain arousal, and relaxation training helps reverse that arousal process.

UNDERSTAND THE CONCENTRATION DEMANDS OF YOUR SPORT

Every sport has different concentration requirements—broad, narrow; deep, shallow; internal, external. For instance, serving in tennis or batting in baseball requires a very narrow external focus, whereas quarterbacking in football, advancing the ball as a point guard in basketball, or club selection in golf require a broad, external focus. Distance swimming and running require a more internal-type focus. Learn to quickly recognize when you're concentrating properly and when you're not. What does it feel like when your concentration is perfect? Where are your eyes? What emotions are present? Practice duplicating the feelings and focus as precisely as possible every time you practice your sport. What you are actually doing with this type of training is improving your control of very specific brain wave patterns.

Take full advantage of naturally occurring breaks during competition for mental recovery and, whenever needed, use such opportunities to refocus and get back on track mentally.

THE MINIMUM NUMBER IS
THIRTY HALF-HOUR SESSIONS

It works like magic, but it does take time. Even with sophisticated EEG neurofeedback equipment, learning to recognize and duplicate IPS neurological patterns, learning how to access and take full advantage of theta states, and learning how to reprogram and recondition yourself through combined relaxation and visualization training require a minimum of twenty to thirty half-hour training sessions.

The question is not whether you can accelerate the learning process but rather *how important* it is in relation to the effort, time, and energy that must be expended. If it's important enough, stay with it for thirty sessions and you'll get significant results.

SUMMARY

From all the available evidence, IPS is essentially a highly specific state of balanced neurological arousal.

Learning concentration skills, understanding the meaning and role of relaxation training, and learning how and when to visualize for maximum effect all relate to controlling the oscillation frequencies of the brain.

IPS, concentration, visualization, and relaxation are intimately interconnected in the context of training brain waves.

Technological advances will clearly change the way that athletes will eventually train mentally to reach their competitive goals. At present, EEG neurofeedback holds great promise. Clearly, the brain is the master organ. Unlocking its vast mysteries should pay significant dividends in every sphere of human pursuit.

EEG research simply confirms what coaches, athletes, and sport psychologists have known for many years. Conclusions like these are just a few examples:

- Athletes concentrate best when they are relaxed and calm.
- Visualization works best when athletes are deeply relaxed.
- Relaxation and visualization are acquired skills that improve with practice.

Most athletes will not have access to EEG neurofeedback equipment. In fact, it's not necessary for accelerated learning. Reaching your best as a competitive athlete can be substantially enhanced by directly training to improve concentration, relaxation, and visualization skills—with or without special biofeedback equipment.

TOUGHNESS TRAINING ASSIGNMENT

1. Tune in to the way you feel when you are concentrating and performing at your best.

Describe in writing how it feels mentally, physically, and emotionally. Make note of things that disrupt your concentration as well as things that help you maintain it: for example, keeping your eyes very controlled.

Pay special attention to feelings of calmness and relaxation during periods of exceptional concentration. Describe feelings of intensity and arousal as you concentrate.

What is the effect of fun and enjoyment on your concentration during competition? What is the effect of fear and anger?

2. Practice some form of relaxation training regularly. Examples include breath control, yoga, meditation, progressive relaxation, and listening to relaxation tapes.

3. Practice visualization daily—both on and off the athletic field. Learn to see, feel, hear, and touch things mentally. Construct as many images of success as you can in your life as an athlete. Use visualization to rehearse your strategies for tomorrow's battles.

4. Combine deep relaxation with visualization and self-suggestion to overcome personal weaknesses. Use a tape with your own voice to reinforce positive themes important to your personal growth. Use short, positive self-statements targeted specifically to your competitive weaknesses. Try to access your theta window. Your target is thirty half-hour practice sessions before significant positive change will be evident.

17

CHALLENGING

YOUR

WEAKNESSES

> Far better it is to dare mighty things, to win glorious triumphs, even though checkered by failure, than to take rank with those poor spirits who neither enjoy much nor suffer much, because they live in the gray twilight that knows not victory nor defeat.
>
> —Theodore Roosevelt

To challenge a weakness is to expose it to stress. Athletes often get so involved in concealing their shortcomings from their competitors that they end up fooling themselves. As you learned in Chapter 7, protecting or hiding from your weaknesses simply perpetuates them.

Two of the most important steps in accelerating the growth process are:

1. Acknowledging that a specific weakness does in fact exist.
2. Devising a strategic plan for systematically exposing the weakness to carefully controlled doses of training stress.

Since this book focuses on both these critical issues, you have learned a great deal about your strengths and weaknesses from the previous chapters. This chapter pulls together all that information so that you can easily formulate a concrete Toughness Training Plan. As you will see, proper goal-setting is one of the most effective ways athletes can target their weaknesses for change.

STRAIGHT ANSWERS TO TOUGH QUESTIONS

Accelerating the toughening process requires straight answers to a number of tough questions. The chapters in this book have been specifically designed to help you formulate solid answers to the following eighteen questions:

1. Based on your composite scores on the CAP, what are your greatest strengths and your greatest weaknesses?

2. How well defined and healthy is your Real Self? What needs associated with your Real Self are not being met? How needy are you? Do you have problems with defensiveness, rigidity, or chronic negativism?

3. Which of the following needs associated with your Real Self should receive your special attention:

a. Food
b. Sleep
c. Rest
d. Safety
e. Self-esteem

4. How effective are your performer skills? Are you a bad actor? How skilled are you in tough acting and tough thinking during competition? What is your Ideal Performance State? What is your "performance script"?

5. To what extent are your competitive problems the result of excessive stress? Is overtraining physically, mentally, or emotionally part of the problem for you? If excessive stress is a problem, what are the primary sources? Parents, coaches, self-imposed pressures?

6. To what extent are your competitive problems the result of too little stress? Have you been overprotected and therefore undertrained? If so, in what specific areas?

7. What are your best markers of overtraining and undertraining? What signals should you look for that indicate stress/recovery imbalance? What are the physical, mental, and emotional symptoms that should signal an alarm for you?

8. What are your most important recovery mechanisms? Do you need to increase the volume of recovery in your total training plan? If so, what are the recovery mechanisms you must improve to achieve your recovery goals? Better diet? Eating more often? More sleep? More naps? Better and more effective episodes of active and passive rest? More humor?

9. Are there recovery opportunities during competition that you can take better advantage of? The four-stage recovery sequence between points in tennis is a good example.

10. What is the meaning for you of negative emotion? How do you differentiate between a need and a want in your training life?

11. How much self-awareness do you have? How great is your capacity for Level I awareness?

12. What is your periodization plan for the next twelve months? When do you want to be at your best? When and how do you intend to make waves throughout the year to achieve your training objectives?

13. What elements of military training can you use to accelerate your toughening process? How can you train to become a more courageous soldier in competition?

14. How physically tough are you? How much abdominal, cardio-respiratory, and generalized muscular stress can you handle? What can you do to prevent future injury? How physically flexible are you?

15. How tough are you mentally? How much mental stress can you handle? How well developed are your positive thinking and visualization skills?

16. What kind of concentration problems do you have during competition? Are you typically over- or underaroused when you compete? What can you do to improve your concentration skills?

17. How effective are your relaxation skills both on and off the athletic field? What's the connection for you between relaxation and concentration? What can you do to improve your relaxation skills?

18. How can you improve your ability to visualize? Do you use visualization to accelerate the learning of motor skills? How can you use visualization to help you overcome stubborn emotional and mental habits that hurt you? What's the connection for you between relaxation and visualization?

EXPOSING YOUR WEAKNESSES TO STRESS

The idea that our muscles become stronger and more resilient when they are exposed to progressively increasing stress is relatively easy for athletes to understand. Applying outside-in stress to accelerate the toughening process is something athletes relate to very quickly. What is not clear in the minds of most athletes is how this toughening principle can be applied to their *mental* and *emotional* weaknesses.

Here's how it works. Remember that stress is energy expenditure. Muscle stress, then, is generated in the process of expending energy. Heavy weights require more energy expenditures than light ones and are, therefore, more stress-producing. Likewise, the greater the number of repetitions, the greater the stress. The important thing here is:

THOUGHTS AND EMOTIONS INVOLVE ENERGY
EXPENDITURES JUST LIKE MUSCLES
DO. EVERY THOUGHT, EVERY IMAGE, EVERY
EMOTION IS A FORM OF STRESS.

Powerful thoughts, images, and emotions are analogous to heavy weights. They require more energy and are therefore more stressful. Repetitiously triggering the same thoughts, images, or emotions is not unlike the repetition of lifting a barbell. Both involve repeated energy expenditure. In the case of such sports as weight lifting, running, cycling, and climbing, growth occurs primarily in the form of muscle adaptations. In the case of thinking, imagery, and emotions, growth occurs primarily in the form of neurological adaptations.

With this understanding, how do you build mental and emotional weaknesses into strengths? How do you attack habits of negative thinking, low self-confidence, impatience, or poor self-discipline?

The first and most important step in converting mental and

emotional weaknesses into strengths is to start expending mental and emotional energy in targeted directions. This becomes a form of mental and emotional practice in the same way motor skills are practiced. Each and every time a thought or image is processed, the adaptation process is stimulated. The more you think a particular thought, the more often you trigger the same image or emotion, the stronger it becomes. Like muscles, the more thoughts, images, and emotions you stimulate, the more accessible they become.

The adaptation process is also influenced by the intensity of the mental or emotional event. Making thoughts and images come alive—with emotion, sounds, colors, and sensations of all kinds—increases energy expenditure and neurological stimulation. And that's the basis of the adaptation process.

Hundreds of repetitions (energy expenditures) are required for a *complex motor skill* to hold up under the pressure of competition. Old bad habits suddenly reappear when motor skills are newly formed or insufficiently practiced. *Mental skills* operate in exactly the same way.

Converting bad habits of thinking to good habits—and turning good habits into strong beliefs—takes time and lots of targeted energy expenditure. Weak thoughts, images, or emotions constantly break down under intense pressure.

The important thing to understand here is that motor skills and mental and emotional skills are acquired in similar ways. Just as targeted repetitions will transform weak motor responses into strong ones, targeted repetition will transform weak thoughts and images into *strong beliefs*.

PRACTICAL EXAMPLES

Weakness: Negative habit of thinking "I hate tie-breakers" as a tennis player.
Consequence: Undermines IPS and results in repeated failure to perform to potential in tie-breakers.

Toughening Process: Exposure to new forms of mental and emotional stress.
What to Do: Any one or a combination of the following could be used to build a new, more adaptive response.

1. Constantly think the affirmation "I love tie-breakers."

2. Repeatedly say to yourself during tie-breakers, "I love it!"

3. Repeatedly visualize performing well in a tie-breaker and loving it. Visualize with strong, positive emotion and enhance the images with sound, colors, and sensations of all kinds.

4. Write about how much you now enjoy tie-breakers—all the reasons why you now enjoy them so much.

5. Combine mental practice with deep relaxation.

Weakness: Lack of discipline on and off the playing field.
Consequence: Contributes to low self-image, constantly interferes with ability to follow training schedules, to follow through on anything.
Toughening Process: Exposure to new forms of mental and emotional stress.
What to Do: Here is a sample plan that could be used to strengthen the capacity for self-discipline.

1. With the coach, list the ten most important things you can do to become more disciplined (targeting stress).

2. Every week focus on successfully fulfilling one of the ten items (applying stress). In ten weeks, all ten items should be implemented.

3. Every week has a new positive theme:

WEEK 1: I'll be on time at practice and class.

WEEK 2: I'll be up by eight a.m. every day except Sunday.

WEEK 3: I'll clean and organize my room and locker daily.

WEEK 4: I'll keep a written daily record that will be checked frequently by my coach.

WEEK 5: I will write a commitment to follow the plan for the upcoming week with an explanation of why this is important.

WEEK 6: I will earn a new nickname from the coach—"Mr. Discipline"—which will be placed on my locker door in big letters.

The keys to success—both in the above examples and in all forms of toughness training—are:

- Positive adaptation and growth requires stress.
- Stress means more targeted energy expenditure.

GOAL-SETTING—THE ART OF TARGETING ENERGY EXPENDITURE

You're now ready to begin rolling out your Toughness Training Plan. Your unique strategic plan will reflect your answers to the eighteen questions presented at the beginning of this chapter. You will also need to reread many of the chapters of this book that relate to your specific needs.

The daily training log in Figure 17.1 is an example of a daily goal-setting chart. It will become the foundation of your Toughness Training Plan.

Here are a few critical principles related to goal-setting:

- Goals are simply targets for energy expenditure. When you set goals you specify how, when, and where you will orchestrate cycles of stress and recovery.

- Always give first priority to targeting your training goals toward overcoming weakness.
- Put your plan down in black and white and put it where you will see it every day.
- Set goals that expose you to stress (pushing you but not leading to overtraining). Listen to your body. Always keep an ear tuned to the language of stress and recovery.
- Center your strategic plan around *performance goals* rather than *outcome goals.*

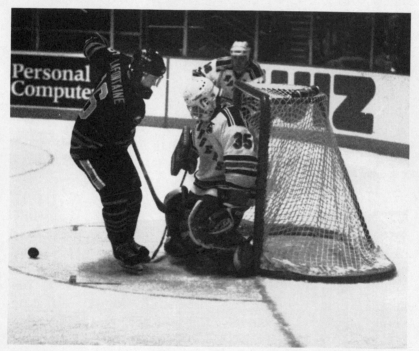

Mike Richter is one of the premier goalies in the NHL. He is noted for his toughness and consistency. In the 1993–1994 season, Mike tied the record for consecutive wins and was the MVP of the All-Star game. Mike began the Toughness Training program in June 1991 and continues to this day.

Performance goals are goals you control absolutely, like doing 200 curl-ups or practicing relaxation skills for ten minutes daily. Outcome goals are goals you don't control absolutely, like winning the tournament, making a particular ranking, or scoring a certain number of points. Outcome goals often backfire. Invest your energies in things you can control and the rest will happen automatically.

- Dream big in the long run; think realistically in the short run.
- It all begins with a dream for the future, and it all happens with what you do today.

Fig. 17.1. Sample for Use in Preparing a Special Form that Meets Your Individual Needs

DAILY TRAINING LOG
(Let Me Count the Waves)

	MON	TUE	WED	THU	FRI	SAT	SUN
1. Interval aerobic exercise (time)							
2. Interval nonaerobic exercise (time)							
3. Curl-ups (no)							
4. Strength training (time)							
5. Stretching (yes/no)							
6. Diet (A–F grade)							
7. Number of meals (often and light)							
8. Quantity of sleep (hours)							
9. Quality of sleep (1–10)							
10. Time to bed/time up							
11. Nap (yes/no)							
12. Visualization practice (time)							
13. Overall volume of stress (1–10)							
14. Quantity of recovery (time)							
15. Quality of recovery (1–10)							
16. Tough thinking (A–F)							
17. Tough acting (A–F)							
18. Patient (A–F)							
19. Independent (A–F)							
20. Stress/recovery balance (1–10)							
21. Felt energy, motivation, fun (1–10)							
22. Disciplined (A–F)							
23. Relaxation tape (time)							
24. How well performed today (1–10)							
25. Got tougher today (yes/no)							

THE IMPORTANCE OF RITUALS

This book and your Toughness Training Plan are designed to help you acquire *the rituals of success.* Repetition of the right physical, mental, and emotional habits eventually brings them under automatic control. Conscious awareness and targeted energy expenditure will gradually give way to automatic rituals of eating, sleeping, resting, stretching, exercising, thinking, acting, recovering, and wave-making that keep you in balance.

Eventually, rituals of success will be put into place that *prepare* you for competition, keep you at peak levels *during* competition, and help you manage your time *after* competition. Every day of toughness training will move you closer to acquiring your own rituals of success.

SUMMARY

The most important questions have been asked, and your answers should be coming in soon. Once they do, a detailed plan of how to expose your weaknesses to training stress should be developed. Create a comprehensive, yet simple and straightforward plan. It is always recommended that athletes start with their weakest links and build from them.

Mental and emotional weaknesses respond to stress in the same way physical weaknesses do. Goal-setting is the vehicle that focuses and directs energy expenditures. A number of guidelines were provided in this chapter to help with the goal-setting process. Designing and following the daily training log represents the core of the toughening process.

TOUGHNESS TRAINING ASSIGNMENT

1. Answer the eighteen questions at the beginning of this chapter the best you can.

2. Develop your own daily training log. Make sure the plan focuses on your specific areas of weakness.

3. Follow the plan daily and make modifications as you learn about yourself and understand your needs better.

18

THE
ENDLESS
JOURNEY

The real voyage of discovery consists not in
seeking new landscapes but in seeing with
new eyes.

—Marcel Proust

An entire career consumed in a single concept—nearly twenty years of searching. So much time but so important. I call it the toughening process—how people grow, how they get stronger and more resilient physically, mentally, and emotionally. At the core is personal courage, the capacity to stand your ground against impossible odds, fearlessly, passionately.

My search for answers took me to the high ground of competitive sport where so much of the battle remains visible, open, testable. And what have I learned? My most important lessons begin and end with "nowhere":

NOWHERE   is the mind-body connection more dramatically visible than in competitive sport. Mind, body, spirit, thoughts, feelings, emotions are all part of the same continuum of life. There is and can be no separation.

NOWHERE   is it more abundantly clear than in competitive sport that everything is interconnected. What you think, how you act, what you eat, how much you sleep, your fighting spirit, your fitness, your passion for life, are all intimately connected.

NOWHERE   is the need for balancing stress and recovery more evident than in competitive sport. The consequences of overtraining and undertraining are painfully clear.

NOWHERE   is it more evident than in competitive sport that, in the long run, toughness prevails over talent every time. Victories in any arena in life will be determined far more by spirit and ability to fight than by genetic gifts.

NOWHERE   is it clearer than in competitive sport that toughness and capacity for fight is formed most powerfully in response to adversity and crisis. It is not the good times, the easy or fun times, that form strength and resiliency in life or sport.

NOWHERE   is it clearer than in competitive sport that every crisis is an opportunity for growth. In life and in sport, stress is the stimulus for growth; during recovery is when you grow. No stress, no growth. No recovery, no growth.

NOWHERE   is it clearer than in competitive sport that you have to love it. Love the grinding, the searching, the pushing, the pulling, the victories, the lessons, the battle itself. And the crazier it gets, the more you have to love it. Becoming the best competitor you can be means loving to compete more than winning. Becoming the best you can be at anything means loving the journey—from beginning to end.

NOWHERE   is it clearer than in competitive sport that you must put yourself on the line every day. You must come totally prepared to fight. You must not turn against yourself during tough times. You must never show weakness. Then and only then will your dreams of total victory take form.

NOWHERE   is it clearer than in competitive sport that the journey into toughness is forever. You never finally arrive, never finally get it, never
finally get over the top. You only get stronger or weaker, closer
or further away; you only grow or don't grow. The objective is to
continue growing, moving forward, challenging yourself to reach
beyond and replace weakness with strength.

NOWHERE   is it clearer than in competitive sport that it's not over till it's
over and that you must *never, never surrender.*

As long as a flicker of life exists, there's hope—hope to fight
back, to rebuild, to grow, to become more, to emerge victorious in
the greatest, most important battle of all—the conquest of self.

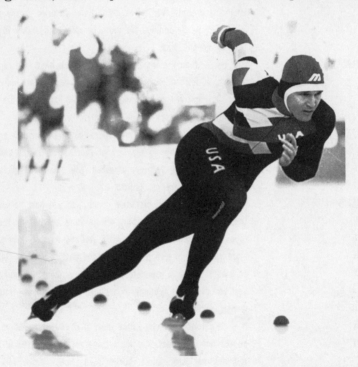

Dan Jansen broke four world records, won two World Cups, a world championship and won the Olympic gold medal, his ultimate dream, using the Toughness Training program. He completed a self-
monitoring Toughness Training Log every day beginning April 1991 and continuing to the present.

APPENDIX: PERIODIC

STRESS/RECOVERY

CHECKS

The following system for checking the balance of stress and recovery uses numbers just as your checkbook does. Rather than tracking dollars, however, you track units of stress and units of recovery.

Clearly, the numbers are only estimates, but experience has shown that this approach can be extremely helpful in understanding and finding balance. This should be done every four to six weeks to sample how you're doing. It is particularly helpful to complete the stress/recovery check during highly stressful times.

Ideally, you match units of recovery with units of stress daily. Realistically, you won't be able to do this every day. When you can't, when your stress scores are quite high compared to your recovery scores for a day or a week, give high priority to increasing your recovery units as soon as possible. A daily stress score of 19 and a recovery score of 17 reflects great balance. Discrepancies of more than three units daily and more than ten units weekly deserve your special attention.

Obviously, chronic overspending leads to trouble. The summary chart enables you to summarize your daily and weekly totals and keep them for quick future reference.

Remember, the closer you get to important competitive events, the more important it is that you build up recovery units. Enter battle fully recovered whenever possible.

STRESS CHECK

1. Quantity of Practice Today_____Hours

2. Intensity of Practice   _____
(How hard you worked)   3,2,1,0

3. Quantity of Competition_____Hours
(Time in competition today)

4. Intensity of Emotional Stress   _____
Associated with Competition   3,2,1,0
(Amount of anger or nervousness experienced before, during, and after competition today)
STRESS: High 3, Medium 2, Low 1, None 0

5. Travel Stress   _____Hours
(Amount of time traveling today)

6. Quantity of Physical Training   _____Hours
(Hours of running, weight lifting, stretching, etc., today)

7. Intensity of Physical Training   _____
(How hard you worked)   3,2,1,0

8. Intensity of Home-Life Stress   _____
(Not sport-related)   3,2,1,0

9. Intensity of Overall Sport Stress   _____
                                                             3,2,1,0

                              _____   _____
                              TOTAL   TOTAL
                              HOURS   INTENSITY
                              (PHYSICAL)   (EMOTIONAL)

_____ + _____ = _____
TOTAL HOURS + TOTAL INTENSITY = TOTAL DAILY STRESS UNITS
(Physical Stress) (Emotional Stress)

RECOVERY CHECK

1. Sleep (Quantity)   _____
   More than 7 hours   = + 4
   5–7 hours   = + 2
   Less than 5 hours   = + .5
2. Sleep (Consistency)   _____
   To bed and up within 30 minutes of normal
   Sleep Time   = + 2
3. Nap   _____
   30 minutes to 1 hour   = + 2
   Less than 30 minutes   = + 1
4. Rest (Active)   _____
   Walking, golf, biking, etc.
   More than 1 hour   = + 2
   30 minutes to 1 hour   = + 1
   Less than 30 minutes   = + .5
5. Rest (Passive)   _____
   Reading, movies, TV, music
   More than 1 hour   = + 2
   30 minutes to 1 hour   = + 1
   Less than 30 minutes   = + .5
6. Relaxation Exercise   _____
   Meditation, breath control, yoga, massage
   More than 1 hour   = + 2
   30 minutes to 1 hour   = + 1
   Less than 30 minutes   = + .5
7. Diet (Number of Meals)   _____
   4 or more light meals   = + 3
   2 to 3 meals   = + 1
8. Diet (Healthy)   _____
   Meals are light, fresh, low-fat, complex-
   carbohydrate centered.
              Yes   = + 3
              Almost   = + 1

9. Fun Times Today
   Feel today was a fun day   = + 2   _____

10. Quantity of Personal Free Time
   1 or more hours   = + 2   _____
   30 minutes to 1 hour   = + 1

                   TOTAL RECOVERY UNITS   _____
                   (MAXIMUM = 24 POINTS)

SUMMARY CHART

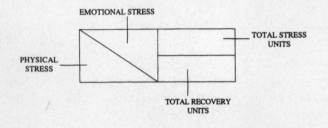

WEEKLY STRESS/RECOVERY SUMMARY
(12 Weeks)

WEEK OF	MON		TUE		WED		THU		FRI		SAT		SUN		TOTAL	

CATEGORIES FOR THE STRESS CHECK

1. Quantity of practice: Record the total hours you spent practicing your sport today (fitness activities are not to be included here).

2. Intensity of practice: Estimate how hard you worked today in your practice using a 0 to 3 scale. A 0 is nothing and a 3 is high intensity.

3. Quantity of competition: Record the total hours you spent competing today. Use the 0 to 3 scale.

4. Intensity of emotional stress associated with competition: Estimate how much stress in the form of negative emotions you experienced before, during, or after competition today. Use the 0 to 3 scale.

5. Travel stress: Record the amount of travel today. Travel is just as stressful as physical training.

6. Quantity of physical training: Record the hours of physical training you did today.

7. Intensity of physical training: Estimate how hard you worked, using the 0 to 3 scale.

8. Intensity of home-life stress: Estimate the intensity of home-life relationships stress in terms of family-related issues. Use the 0 to 3 scale.

9. Intensity of overall sport stress: Estimate the overall emotional stress associated with sport. Use the 0 to 3 scale.

CATEGORIES FOR THE RECOVERY CHECK

Ten categories are used in estimating the total volume of recovery for a twenty-four-hour period. They are all self-explanatory and therefore will not be listed here. The maximum number of recovery units you can earn in a twenty-four-hour period is twenty-four.

When convenient, simply transfer the totals to the summary chart included in this Appendix. It has space for twelve weeks.

RECOMMENDED
READING

BRENNAN, RICHARD. *The Alexander Technique Workbook*. Rockport: Element, 1992.

CLARK, NANCY. *Sports Nutrition Guidebook*. Champaign, IL: Leisure Press, 1990.

CSIKSZENTMIHALYI, MIHALY. *Flow*. New York: Harper & Row, 1991.

FLECK, STEVEN and KRAEMER, WILLIAM. *Designing Resistance Training Programs*. Champaign, IL: Human Kinetics, 1987.

GROPPEL, JACK and KNIGHT, LES. *Sports Nutrition: The "Get Tough" Book*. Lakeland, FL: Knight, 1993.

GROPPEL, JACK; LOEHR, JAMES; MELVILLE, SCOTT; and QUINN, ANN. *Science of Coaching Tennis*. Champaign, IL: Leisure Press, 1989.

HUTCHISM, MICHAEL. *Mega Brain*. New York: Ballantine, 1991.

KELEMAN, STANLEY. *Emotional Anatomy*. Berkeley: Center Press, 1985.

LOEHR, JAMES. *Toughness Training for Life*. New York: Plume, 1994.
———. *The Mental Game*. New York: Plume, 1990.

————. *Mental Toughness Training for Sports*. New York: Plume, 1987.

MOYERS, BILL. *Healing and the Mind*. New York: Doubleday, 1993.

MURPHY, MICHAEL. *The Future of the Body*. New York: Putnam, 1993.

PELLETIER, KENNETH. *Mind as Healer, Mind as Slayer*. New York: Dell, 1992.

ROSSI, EARNEST. *The 20 Minute Break*. Los Angeles: Jeremy Tarcher, 1991.

WALTON, GARY. *Beyond Winning*. Champaign, IL: Leisure Press, 1992.

INDEX